Get Through MRCOG Part 2

Get Through MRCOG Part 2

EMQs

Second Edition

Kalaivani Ramalingam, DGO, FRCOG, CCT (UK), PgC
(Medical Education)
UroGynaecologist and Obstetrician
Apollo Hospitals
Chennai, India

Latha Mageswari Palanivelu, DGO, FRCOG (UK), DFFP (UK)
Consultant Obstetrician and Gynaecologist
Dr. Rela Institute and Medical Centre
Chennai, India

Lakshmi Thirumalaikumar, MD, FRCOG, MSc (Diabetes)
Consultant Obstetrician
Birmingham City Hospital
Birmingham, United Kingdom

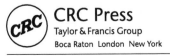
CRC Press
Taylor & Francis Group
Boca Raton London New York

CRC Press is an imprint of the
Taylor & Francis Group, an **informa** business

CRC Press
Taylor & Francis Group
6000 Broken Sound Parkway NW, Suite 300
Boca Raton, FL 33487-2742

© 2020 by Taylor & Francis Group, LLC
CRC Press is an imprint of Taylor & Francis Group, an Informa business

No claim to original U.S. Government works

Printed on acid-free paper

International Standard Book Number-13: 978-0-367-34051-3 (Hardback)
978-1-138-19777-0 (Paperback)

Visit the Taylor & Francis Web site at
http://www.taylorandfrancis.com

and the CRC Press Web site at
http://www.crcpress.com

Contents

CONTENTS

CONTENTS

Editors

Kalaivani Ramalingam is a senior obstetrician and urogynaecologist at Apollo Hospitals, Chennai, India. She has had an interest in postgraduate medical education, particularly the Mid-Region Council of Governments (MRCOG) exam preparation since her early days of training. She completed her Certificate of Completion of Training (CCT) course at Wessex Deanery and worked as a substantive National Health Service (NHS) consultant in Kingston upon Thames between 2011 and 2014 before returning to her home country of India. She continues to pursue her academic interests, particularly in urogynaecology.

Latha Mageswari Palanivelu is a consultant and clinical lead in obstetrics and gynaecology, working at the Dr. Rela Institute and Medical Centre, Chennai. Her special interests are high-risk obstetrics and perinatal medicine. Trained in India and the UK, she regularly participates in academic activities.

Lakshmi Thirumalaikumar is a consultant obstetrician with a special interest in maternal medicine and diabetes. She has worked as a consultant obstetrician in the West Midlands region for more than ten years. She is passionate about teaching and training. Her contribution towards postgraduate training has been well appreciated by the specialty trainees.

Introduction

Great things happen when ideas are put to work.

Congratulations on passing Part 1 of the MRCOG exam. This is possibly why this book is being explored by you to obtain information on preparation for the Part 2 exam.

As most trainees are aware, the MRCOG exam now consists of three parts. After passing Part 1, Part 2 tests the clinical application of knowledge obtained at the fifth-year specialist training level or ST5. It is essential to pass the MRCOG exam in order to proceed to the advanced years of training in ST6. The exam aims to assess the trainees' fitness to progress in their training and their knowledge basis.

The MRCOG exam is also a popular exam outside the United Kingdom. Many practitioners from around the world have been attempting the exam and have been successful with adequate preparation and awareness of the training system in the United Kingdom.

General information

The Part 2 MRCOG exam usually takes place at least twice a year. Exam centres may vary in some locations. The information on upcoming exam centres is provided during the application process and is available on the website of the Royal College of Obstetricians and Gynaecologists (RCOG) and is updated constantly. UK centres are usually at London, Manchester, Edinburgh and Dublin.

Many international centres are also exam venues and are available in the following countries:

- Bangladesh
- Egypt
- Hong Kong
- India (Bangalore, Delhi)
- Iraq
- Myanmar
- Oman
- Pakistan (Lahore)
- Saudi Arabia (Riyadh)
- Singapore
- Sudan

- UAE (Abu Dhabi)
- West Indies (Trinidad)

Purpose of the book

The purpose of this book is to enable trainees preparing for the Part 2 MRCOG exam to get adequate practice in the extended matching questions (EMQs) format of the exam. The Part 2 MRCOG exam is currently a written exam. A prerequisite is passing the Part 1 exam and having a satisfactory assessment of the requisite training, as stated on the website of the RCOG.

The assessment of training is mandatory before applying for the Part 2 exam. Adequate time must be given (at least 6 weeks) for the college to assess completed forms. The information and forms are available in the requisite section of the RCOG website.

The current format of the exam comprises two written papers. The time allowed for each paper is 3 hours, and each paper consists of 50 EMQs and 50 single best answers (or SBAs, for short). The EMQs are more extensive and take longer to answer. Of the total marks, 60% is allotted to the EMQs and 40% to the SBAs. The RCOG recommends a time management of 110 minutes for the EMQs and 70 minutes for the SBAs in each paper. There is a much-needed break of one hour in between the two exam papers.

Preparation for the exam

The syllabus is vast, comprising the entirety of clinical obstetrics and gynaecology. For practical purposes, the syllabus has been devised in line with the modules for the specialty training (ST) in the United Kingdom. This gives the candidate an exhaustive though defined list of topics required for the knowledge base prior to the exam.

It is very important to note that this is a clinically oriented exam. But for an occasional statistics or basic science theory question, the emphasis is on clinical decision-making and appropriate management given the circumstances in question.

More than cramming knowledge, revision of questions exposes a candidate to many different scenarios and widens the thought process. The revision resources are clearly outlined in the RCOG part 2 exam resources page.

The RCOG website (www.rcog.org.uk) remains the best resource per se for exam preparation along with its green top guidelines, patient information sheets, scientific impact papers, standard terminology (STRATOG) and The Obstetrician and Gynaecologist (TOG) articles.

How is an EMQ different from other exam assessment tools?

The EMQ paper in the exam comprises a separate question paper with 50 EMQs and an answer sheet numbered 1–50. Each EMQ question starts with an option list between A and T. This is followed by a lead-in statement explaining what the requirement for the question is, for example, management or diagnosis, next appropriate step, and so on. This is followed by questions on the topic, usually 3–5.

The answer sheet has A–T lozenges for each question between 1 and 20. The option list typically has at least 10 answers in each list. Each answer carries a mark, and there is no negative marking or penalising for wrong answers.

Top tips for EMQ

- *Read the lead-in statement first.* This helps to know what is required for answering each question in that segment.
- *Do not* read the option list first. This leads to unnecessary confusion about possible questions and generates anxiety.
- *Read each question slowly,* and find a plausible answer in your mind, and then find the closest response from the option list. This is where a good knowledge base and adequate practice of questions help.
- *Do not* spend a lot of time on ambiguous or unknown EMQs. Return to questions that you find difficult after answering easier questions.
- *Remember* to mark the responses in the right space on the answer sheet, especially if you jump the question order.
- *Check* the answer sheet at the end for appropriate intended answers and be sure that only one lozenge has been shaded for each EMQ question.
- *Do not panic* looking at the entirety of the EMQ paper.
- *Remember,* if it is a difficult question for you to answer as a well-prepared candidate, it is difficult for every other candidate, too!
- *Nothing* works but consistent practice and revision for the exam.
- *Familiarise* yourself with the clinical practice in the United Kingdom if you are an overseas candidate.

Chapter 1: Obstetric EMQs

1.1 Preconception counselling

Options:

A advice against pregnancy
B advice regarding diet, nutrition and exercise
C cessation of smoking and lifestyle modification
D complete blood count, HbA1c, blood sugar and renal function tests
E complete blood count, screening for asymptomatic bacteriuria
F genetic counselling
G lifestyle advice and high-dose folic acid supplement
H omega fatty acids supplement
I partner screening
J preconceptional folic acid
K prophylactic antibiotics
L prophylactic cervical cerclage
M rubella screening and 400 mcg folic acid daily
N screening for sexually transmitted infections
O uterine artery Doppler study

For each of the following questions, choose the *single*-most appropriate option from the list A–O. Each option may be chosen once, more than once or not at all.

Questions:

1 A 34-year-old Asian woman attends the preconception clinic for advice before planning her pregnancy. She weighs 98 kg and her BMI is 35. She is known to have type 1 diabetes mellitus and is on treatment with insulin. Her recent blood sugar levels are within normal limits. Her HbA1c is 5.2%.

2 A 28-year-old Caucasian woman is contemplating pregnancy. She had donated her kidney to her twin brother a year ago. She is a non-smoker with a BMI of 24. She is Rubella immune.

3 A 42-year-old woman seeks preconception advice. She smokes 15 cigarettes a day and is on medication for chronic obstructive airway disease. She does not have any respiratory difficulty at rest, and a recent echocardiogram reveals moderate pulmonary hypertension.

4 A 29-year-old banker seeks advice regarding pregnancy. She is healthy and smokes socially. She was never in a long-term relationship and was screened negative for STIs recently.

5 A 27-year-old woman attends the outpatient clinic for advice. She was diagnosed with severe post-partum psychosis and continues to be stable on clozapine. She regularly attends counselling sessions regularly and is on follow-up with the psychiatric team.

For answers, see 2.1.

1.2 Management of early pregnancy

Options:

A   commence low-dose aspirin
B   commence low-molecular-weight heparin and low-dose aspirin
C   immediate catheterisation and reassurance
D   inpatient HDU care with hydration, analgesia and observation
E   intramuscular 17 OH progesterone injections
F   intramuscular methotrexate followed by folinic acid
G   intravenous access and urgent pelvic ultrasonography
H   laparoscopic salpingectomy
I   MSU culture followed by intravenous antibiotics
J   offer detailed counselling about selective termination
K   oral progesterone
L   prophylactic antibiotics
M   reassurance
N   serial serum beta-hCG levels
O   termination of pregnancy

For each of the following questions, choose the *single*-most appropriate intervention option from the list A–O. Each option may be chosen once, more than once or not at all.

Questions:

1   A 26-year-old woman presents to the A & E with fever, vomiting and severe pain in her abdomen and flank. The last menstrual period was 6 weeks ago. Her urine pregnancy test is positive and urinalysis shows multiple pus cells and epithelial cells. On examination, she is found to be dehydrated with a pulse of 98 beats per minute (bpm), and her blood pressure (BP) is 80/40 mmHg with rigidity and guarding in the pelvic region.

2   A 16-year-old student attends the early pregnancy unit with mild abdominal pain and not being able to pass urine for the past 12 hours. A recent ultrasound examination showed a viable intrauterine singleton pregnancy. On examination her vital signs are found to be stable with lower abdominal distension.

3   A 33-year-old primigravida presents to the early pregnancy unit at 10-week gestation with painful vaginal bleeding. On examination, her vital signs are found to be stable. Speculum examination reveals mild vaginal bleeding with a closed cervix. Ultrasound examination shows a viable intrauterine pregnancy. Her urinalysis is normal.

4   A 37-year-old woman presents to her GP with 6 weeks of amenorrhoea. She undergoes an ultrasound examination in the early pregnancy unit and is found to have a heterotopic pregnancy without cardiac activity in the ectopic sac. She is completely asymptomatic with stable vital signs.

5   A 36-year-old woman is referred from the radiology department after her dating scan with a spontaneous, viable 7-week quadruplet pregnancy. She has mild dysuria and abdominal pain. Examination shows PR of 78 bpm and BP of 110/70 mmHG with a normal abdominal examination.

For answers, see 2.2.

1.3 Infections in pregnancy

Options:

A   antiviral therapy and HDU care
B   category 3 lower segment Caesarean section
C   catheterisation and oral antibiotics
D   combined vaccination and immunisation (active and passive)
E   high dependency care with intravenous antibiotics and hydration
F   immediate laparotomy
G   induction of labour
H   intramuscular betamethasone 12 mg 12 hours apart
I   MRI abdomen and pelvis
J   oral acyclovir 400 mg three times daily for 5 days
K   oral acyclovir 800 mg five times daily for 7 days
L   reassurance
M   serum antibody testing varicella IgG and IgM
N   urine routine analysis and midstream culture
O   varicella zoster immunoglobulin (VZIG) administration

For each of the following questions, choose the *single*-most appropriate option from the list A–O. Each option may be chosen once, more than once or not at all.

Questions:

1   A 28-year-old woman presents to the A & E at 30 weeks gestation with fever, flank pain and palpitations. On examination, she is found to be febrile with pulse rate (PR) 100 bpm and BP 100/60 mmHG. She has diffuse tenderness over the abdomen with soft, non-tender uterus. Vaginal examination is normal and the fetal heart rate is found to be 200 bpm.

2   A 30-year-old woman presents to the early pregnancy assessment unit with difficulty in passing urine at 12 weeks gestation. She denies any fever, dysuria or vaginal bleeding. On examination, she is found to have shallow painful ulcers over the perineum.

3   A 21-year-old woman presents to the early pregnancy assessment unit at 9-week gestation with fever and vesicular generalised rashes of 3 days duration. There is no difficulty in breathing or neck stiffness. Clinical examination shows a PR of 96 bpm and BP of 110/60 mmHG.

4   A 20-year-old primigravida presents at term +4 to the delivery suite for induction of labour. She perceives fetal movements well and obstetric ultrasonogram is normal. On examination, she is noted to have painful ulcers over the perineum. She denies any difficulty in passing urine or facing similar episodes in the past.

5 An 18-year-old girl presents to the A & E with watery vaginal discharge. She is found to be 32 weeks pregnant. She had not returned to the obstetric unit after her initial visit in early pregnancy. Her uterus is contracting mildly. On vaginal examination, her cervix is found to be partially effaced with clear liquor draining. Ultrasound shows a normally grown fetus with adequate liquor. Her blood results are positive for HBsAg and negative for anti-HCV antibodies. Liver function tests are within normal limits.

For answers, see 2.3.

1.4 Antenatal screening I

Options:

A   amniocentesis and FISH test
B   blood sugar levels fasting and postprandial, HbA1C levels
C   chorionic villi sampling
D   expectant management
E   folic acid and iron supplementation
F   genetic counselling
G   genetic testing of mother for carrier status
H   maternal blood test of fetal cells
I   partner screening
J   polymerase chain reaction (PCR) of fetal DNA from amniotic cells
K   preimplantation genetic testing
L   reassurance
M   second trimester serum screening
N   serial obstetric Doppler studies
O   termination of pregnancy
P   three-dimensional ultrasound
Q   umbilical cord blood sampling

For each of the following questions, choose the *single*-most appropriate option from the list A–Q. Each option may be chosen once, more than once or not at all.

Questions:

1   A 26-year-old Greek woman attends the antenatal clinic at 8 week of gestation with her early pregnancy scan report. She is known to have sickle cell disease (HbSS) and is being followed up adequately. Her partner is from the same ethnic background with HbSC.

2   A 26-year-old primigravida undergoes an anomaly scan at 20 weeks, which shows echogenic bowel loops. Her integrated screening test result was negative. Both parents subsequently undergo evaluation and both are found to be cystic fibrosis (CF) mutant gene positive.

3   A 20-year-old student of Asian origin attends the antenatal clinic for advice. She is very pale and further evaluation shows her haemoglobin to be 8.6 g/dL with MCV 70 fL. Electrophoresis shows alpha thalassemia to be minor.

4   A 28-year-old woman of Mediterranean background attends the antenatal clinic at 12 weeks gestation with low-risk combined screening test result. Two of her relatives have been diagnosed with Duchenne muscular dystrophy and seeks your advice.

For answers, see 2.4.

1.5 Antenatal screening II

Options:

A   amniocentesis and FISH test
B   blood sugar levels fasting and postprandial, HbA1C levels
C   chorionic villi sampling
D   genetic counselling
E   genetic screening for the couple
F   maternal blood test of fetal cells
G   obstetric Doppler studies
H   partner genetic screening
I   postnatal ultrasound
J   reassurance
K   screening single-gene disorder
L   second trimester serum screening
M   third trimester serial growth scans
N   three-dimensional ultrasound
O   umbilical cord blood sampling

For each of the following questions, choose the *single*-most appropriate option from the list A–O. Each option may be chosen once, more than once or not at all.

Questions:

1   A 24-year-old primigravida undergoes target scan at 21 weeks gestation, which shows bilateral choroid plexus cysts. No other problems are noted. Her first trimester combined screening is negative.

2   A 37-year-old second gravida is seen at the antenatal clinic at 20 weeks gestation. Her ultrasound report shows femur length shorter than third centile, with no other abnormalities. Her first trimester integrated test was normal.

3   A 26-year-old third gravida with two previous mid-trimester miscarriages is being reviewed at 12 weeks gestation with her ultrasound report. Nuchal translucency is reported as 4.6 mm.

4   A 30-year-old lady is attending the antenatal clinic with target scan report, which shows bilateral renal pelviectasis with no other abnormalities. Right side measures 7 mm and left side is 8.6 mm. Her previous screening reports and other parameters are normal.

For answers, see 2.5.

1.6 Preterm labour/PPROM

Options:

A betamethasone, 12 mg 24 hours apart
B category I lower segment Caesarean section
C cervical length assessment by ultrasound
D commence magnesium sulfate regimen
E emergency cervical cerclage
F fetal fibronectin assay
G high vaginal swab for bacterial culture
H *in utero* transfer
I indomethacin 100 mg per rectal once 24 hours
J intravenous Atosiban 6.75 mg over 1-minute bolus followed by infusion
K intravenous benzylpenicillin
L MSU culture and urine routine analysis
M oral erythromycin and betamethasone
N oral nifedipine 20 mg followed by 10–20 mg four doses in 24 hours
O ritodrine infusion

For each of the following questions, choose the *single*-most appropriate option from the list A–O. Each option may be chosen once, more than once or not at all.

Questions:

1 A 38-year-old second gravida with previous normal delivery at term presents at 26 weeks gestation with leaking vaginal. She denies any pain or bleeding and examination shows a soft non-tender uterus with no cervical changes. Pooling of liquor is seen in the posterior fornix. Her antenatal period was otherwise normal and anomaly scan was also normal.

2 A 33-year-old primigravida attends the DAU at 33 weeks gestation complaining of abdominal pain and leaking vaginal. On examination, she is noted to have regular uterine contractions with partially effaced cervix.

3 A 22-year-old third gravida presents at 29-week gestation with leaking vaginal. On examination, she is found to have regular uterine contractions, and her fetus is felt in the transverse position. Cervix is found to be 4 cm dilated.

4 A 20-year-old primigravida attends the day assessment unit at 23 weeks gestation with increased vaginal discharge and abdominal discomfort. Abdominal examination confirms a soft non-tender uterus, and vaginal examination reveals a soft cervix with no bleeding or draining. Transvaginal scan shows a cervix of 1.5 cm length.

5 A 26-year-old woman presents to the delivery suite with painful contractions and vaginal bleeding. She is currently 35 weeks pregnant and abdominal examination shows a tense uterus with an uneffaced cervix and vaginal bleeding.

For answers, see 2.6.

1.7 Post-partum haemorrhage I

Options:

A   activated factor 7
B   bimanual compression
C   brace sutures (B-Lynch suture)
D   examination under anaesthesia
E   foley's catheter, maternal observation including output
F   internal iliac ligation
G   intra-abdominal packing
H   intrauterine balloon
I   intravenous colloids
J   laparotomy/hysterectomy and proceed
K   manual removal of placenta under general anaesthesia
L   oral/rectal misoprostol 800 mcg
M   prostaglandin F2α
N   resuscitation with two wide-bore cannula, complete blood count and coagulation profile U&Es and cross-match 6 units of blood
O   secure airway and 100% oxygen
P   syntocinon 40 units in 500 mL infusion
Q   uterine artery embolization

For each of the following questions, choose the *single*-most appropriate option from the list A–Q. Each option may be chosen once, more than once or not at all.

Questions:

1   A 34-year-old woman collapses in the day assessment unit. She was complaining about heavy bleeding since morning. She had been discharged from the hospital the day before following spontaneous vaginal delivery. On examination, she is found to be unconscious and her BP is 60/40 mmHG, she has weak PR and her respiratory rate is 36 per minute.

2   A 36-year-old woman is undergoing lower segment Caesarean section following a failed forceps delivery under general anaesthesia. Following delivery of the baby, a PPH is noted during laparotomy. After responding initially to uterotonics, the uterus is atonic with profuse bleeding. Blood and volume expanders have been requested. Patient is now haemodynamically stable.

3   Severe PPH is encountered in a 29-year-old woman after spontaneous vertex delivery. Placenta and membranes have been expelled. Baby weighs 8 pounds with good APGAR score. After shifting from the delivery suite, the midwife notes vaginal bleeding more than usual. Her BP is 100/60 mmHG. PR is 98 bpm. On examination, her uterus was found to be relaxing in between and responding very well to oxytocin infusion.

4   Following a forceps delivery, a 36-year-old-parous woman has profuse vaginal bleeding. Uterus is well contracted with no signs of placental separation. Immediate resuscitative measures are taken.

5   A 30-year-old multiparous woman has precipitate labour and quick delivery in A & E. She is noted to have atonic uterus with a deep perineal tear and profuse vaginal bleeding. Her intravenous access is secured and blood products has been arranged.

For answers, see 2.7.

1.8 Post-partum haemorrhage II

Options:

A B-Lynch suture
B balloon tamponade
C bimanual compression
D examination under anaesthesia
E foley's catheter and fluid balance
F internal iliac ligation
G intra-abdominal/pelvic packing
H intramuscular carboprost 0.25 mg
I intramuscular ergometrine 0.5 mg
J intravenous crystalloids
K laparotomy/hysterectomy and proceed
L manual removal under general anaesthesia
M oral/rectal misoprostol 1000 mcg
N secure airway and 100% oxygen
O slow intravenous oxytocin 5 units
P two wide-bore cannula, CBC, coagulation profile, U & Es and cross-match 6 units of blood
Q uterine artery embolization

For each of the following questions, choose the *single*-most appropriate option from the list A–Q. Each option may be chosen once, more than once or not at all.

Questions:

1 A 32-year-old woman undergoes an elective Caesarean section for previous C-section with intrauterine growth restriction. Following delivery of the fetus, uterus is tonic but placenta is found to be morbidly adherent with no clear plane of separation. All the prerequisites had been arranged already as placenta accreta was suspected in the earlier scan.

2 A 27-year-old woman delivers a 9-pound baby by vacuum extraction at term. At 5 minutes with continuous cord traction, a shaggy mass comes out of the vagina with the placenta still *in situ*. The problem is recognised immediately and the uterus is replaced. The uterus is atonic with profuse bleeding encountered subsequently. The patient's PR is 100 bpm and BP is 80/40 mmHG.

3 A 24-year-old primigravida undergoes induction of labour at 35 weeks gestation for severe preeclampsia. She is on magnesium sulfate regimen for the past 18 hours. After spontaneous delivery, she has post-partum haemorrhage for which she is given oxytocin injection and rectal misoprostol.

For answers, see 2.8.

1.9 Acute intrapartum events

Options:

A   call for help
B   cardiopulmonary resuscitation
C   category I LSCS
D   delivery of posterior shoulder
E   documentation with care
F   evaluate the episiotomy
G   external cephalic version
H   immediate intubation and 100% oxygen
I   internal podalic version followed by breech extraction
J   McRoberts manoeuvre
K   perimortem Caesarean delivery
L   secure airway, oxygen breathing and circulation
M   start oxytocin infusion 5 units in 500 mL of Hartman's solution
N   suprapubic pressure
O   Trendelenburg position and bladder filling

For each of the following questions, choose the *single*-most appropriate option from the list A–O. Each option may be chosen once, more than once or not at all.

Questions:

1   A 27-year-old third gravida presents at 38-week gestation to the obstetric day care unit with leaking vaginal. On examination, she is noted to have mild contractions. Fetal heart rate is 140 bpm. Vaginal examination shows a soft pulsatile mass in the vagina.

2   A 30-year-old lady is being induced at 10 days post-term. She has a forceps delivery under epidural anaesthesia. Thirty seconds following the delivery of the head, difficulty is encountered.

3   A 24-year-old-parous woman has a spontaneous water birth at term. After 5 minutes, profuse bleeding is noted and a big mass is noted at the introitus. The mother then becomes unconscious.

4   A 30-year-old woman is labouring in her second pregnancy at 38 weeks gestation. Her first pregnancy was a planned Caesarean section for breech presentation. Epidural pain relief is given and she is being monitored by continuous cardiotocography. She has good uterine contractions and vaginal examination done an hour ago showed 6 cm dilated cervix with vertex at −3 station. Sudden bradycardia to 82 bpm lasting for 2 minutes is noted.

5   A 24-year-old woman is noted to throw tonic-clonic convulsions when she attends the delivery suite. She is a primigravida at 30 weeks gestation and is being monitored in the antenatal ward for pre-eclampsia.

For answers, see 2.9.

1.10 Maternal collapse I

Options:

A   call for help
B   CT pulmonary angiogram
C   documentation
D   external cephalic version
E   high dependency unit admission, hydration, supportive care
F   initial stabilisation and Category 1 Caesarean section
G   initiate magnesium sulfate regime
H   initiate sliding scale insulin protocol
I   IV heparin infusion
J   laparotomy after initial stabilisation
K   MRI brain
L   perimortem Caesarean section
M   secure airway and 100% oxygen, and intravenous access
N   two wide-bore cannula, CBC, coagulation profile U & Es and cross-match
O   uterine relaxant (halothane)

For each of the following questions, choose the *single*-most appropriate option from the list A–O. Each option may be chosen once, more than once or not at all.

Questions:

1   A 34-year-old woman is being transported by an ambulance to the A & E in a collapsed state 6 days after a normal delivery. Her hospital course prior to discharge was uneventful. On examination, she is found to have a feeble pulse but no recordable BP.

2   A 30-year-old woman, on second post-operative day following a Caesarean section for failed induction, complains of severe myalgia and headache. She is dehydrated, febrile with a temperature of 104°F and shows signs of cerebral irritability. Diffuse tenderness is noted across lower abdomen with a contracted uterus.

3   A 26-year-old primigravida at 36 weeks gestation is seen at A & E with complaints of confusion and palpitation. She is a known type 1 diabetic and is on insulin. Examination reveals dehydration, tachycardia and tachypnoea. Urine examination shows ketonuria.

4   A 28-year-old in her third pregnancy is rushed to hospital emergency in a state of collapse. She is a known smoker at 32 week of gestation. She had earlier complained of severe abdominal pain. Abdominal examination shows a rigid uterus with fetal heart rate of 100 bpm. Initial resuscitative measures have been done.

5   A primigravida is being induced at 2 weeks post-term. She is on oxytocin infusion, and fetal heartbeat is being monitored continuously. Last examination showed 5 cm dilatation with a bag of membranes which was ruptured. Liquor was clear. She complains of severe chest pain and breathing difficulty. Her PR is 102 bpm and BP is 90/60 mmHG.

For answers, see 2.10.

1.11 Maternal collapse II

Options:

A ABC-check airway, breathing and oxygen, and intravenous access
B call for help
C coronary angiography
D CT pulmonary angiogram
E documentation
F high dependency unit admission, hydration, supportive care
G initial stabilization and lower segment Caesarean section
H initiate magnesium sulfate regime
I initiate sliding scale insulin protocol
J intravenous heparin loading dose followed by infusion
K laparotomy after initial stabilisation
L MRI brain
M perimortem Caesarean section
N two wide-bore cannula, CBC, coagulation profile U & Es and cross-match
O uterine relaxant (halothane)

For each of the following questions, choose the *single*-most appropriate option from the list A–O. Each option may be chosen once, more than once or not at all.

Questions:

1 An 18-year-old primigravida at 28 weeks gestation presents to her GP with a history of giddiness. She suddenly collapses at the GP surgery and her initial resuscitation is done. She is being transported to the hospital. She is known to have a history of substance abuse.

2 A 38-year-old woman attends the postnatal clinic for review. She smokes 10 cigarettes a day and has been experiencing sharp chest pain accompanied by sweating and palpitations. Her PR is 110 bpm with a BP of 90/60 mmHG. Her ECG shows ST segment elevation. She has been transferred to the high dependency unit and is in a stable condition.

3 A 23-year-old woman with known rheumatic heart disease complains of weakness and numbness over her left arm. She is currently 10 weeks pregnant and is on thromboprophylaxis for a replaced mitral valve. She has stable vital signs.

4 A 29-year-old second gravida undergoes amniocentesis at 18 weeks gestation for high-risk serum Down's syndrome test. During the procedure, she complains of chest tightness and breathing difficulty and becomes unconscious.

For answers, see 2.11.

1.12 Domestic violence

Options:

A   arranging a translator to be in attendance
B   call for help and start basic life support
C   counselling
D   documentation verbatim
E   emergency contraception IUCD
F   emergency contraception levonorgestrel 1.5 g stat
G   enquiring and training the staff concerned
H   immediate hospitalisation
I   inform police
J   involvement of senior clinician at delivery is needed for anterior episiotomy
K   liaise with social services
L   postexposure prophylaxis for HIV and continued sexual health follow-up
M   psychiatrist involvement
N   referral to genitourinary clinic (GUM) clinic
O   seek trust lawyer's advice
P   sexual assault and referral centre

For each of the following questions, choose the *single*-most appropriate option from the list A–P. Each option may be chosen once, more than once or not at all.

Questions:

1   An 18-year-old third gravida with no live births complains of frequent urinary infections. She is found to be 12 weeks pregnant. She had earlier been prescribed a course of antibiotics, and a recent ultrasound was normal. Culture has always been negative.

2   A 15-year-old girl is seen in the A & E for urinary retention. She is noted to be 20 weeks pregnant with purulent vaginal discharge.

3   A 16-year-old girl presents at term gestation to the antenatal clinic. She has not been to any antenatal service so far. She is accompanied by her partner and does not speak English.

4   A 30-year-old woman at 28 weeks gestation presents to her GP with vulval lesions. She had been treated for genitourinary infections in the past. On examination, extensive herpetic lesions were noted.

5   A 20-year-old woman of Afro-Caribbean origin is seen in the delivery suite with complaints of watery vaginal discharge. She is 36 weeks pregnant. On examination, it was found that she had extensive labial adhesions.

6   A 30-year-old woman presents to the A & E with a history of fall. She is 30 weeks pregnant. She was examined earlier in the antenatal clinic twice in the same week with abdominal discomfort and weakness. She is noted to have bruises all over her body. Her general and obstetric parameters are normal.

For answers, see 2.12.

1.13 Thromboembolism in pregnancy

Options:

A cava filters
B change to low-molecular-weight heparin
C commence low-molecular-weight heparin – enoxaparin 1.5 mg/kg body weight
D commence warfarin
E CTPA-Computerised tomography pulmonary angiogram
F D-dimer testing
G duplex ultrasound
H ECG and chest X-ray
I heparin infusion
J hydration and TED stockings
K initial resuscitation, and basic blood FBC, coagulation profile and liver function tests
L low-dose aspirin (75 mg)
M peak anti-Xa level
N prophylactic low-molecular-weight heparin enoxaparin 40 mg once daily
O spiral computed tomography pulmonary angiography (CT-PA)
P ventilation/perfusion (V/Q) scanning

For each of the following questions, choose the *single*-most appropriate option from the list A–P. Each option may be chosen once, more than once or not at all.

Questions:

1 A 28-year-old primigravida presents to the A & E at 16 weeks gestation with chest pain and breathlessness. She smokes 15 cigarettes a day and has not seen her midwife or GP yet for her pregnancy booking. On examination she is found to be very pale, dyspnoeic with a PR of 112 bpm and respiratory rate of 30 pm. She is clinically stable and is admitted to the high dependency unit.

2 A 33-year-old second gravida attends the (DAU) day assessment unit with a dull ache in her calf region at 22 weeks gestation. She has no other symptoms. On examination, it was found that she had tenderness in her calf. Duplex study shows a deep vein thrombus.

3 A 24-year-old woman attends the antenatal clinic at 8 weeks gestation for further care. She is known to have protein S deficiency and is currently on warfarin.

4 A 28-year-old woman is being induced for gestational diabetes at 37 completed weeks of gestation. She weighs 78 kg and her sugar levels are well controlled with insulin. She undergoes an emergency Caesarean section for fetal distress. The agent of choice for thromboprophylaxis is … .

5 A 37-year-old postnatal mother presents with calf pain. She is diagnosed with recurrent DVT and receives therapeutic dose of low-molecular-weight heparin. She is otherwise well not stable. Further evaluation shows a right common iliac vein thrombus.

For answers, see 2.13.

1.14 Hypertensive disorders in pregnancy

Options:

A admission to high dependency unit and supportive care
B airway, face mask oxygen and intravenous access
C betamethasone 12 mg two doses
D blood investigation CBC, urea and electrolytes, creatinine, LFT and uric acid
E category I Caesarean section
F catheterisation and strict fluid management
G commence oral labetalol
H computerised tomography of brain
I *in utero* transfer
J intravenous calcium administration
K intravenous hydralazine 10 mg bolus followed by maintenance
L intravenous magnesium sulphate 4 g bolus followed by 1 g per hour
M oral/sublingual nifedipine 10 mg
N thromboprophylaxis with enoxaparin

For each of the following questions, choose the *single*-most appropriate management option from the list A–N. Each option may be chosen once, more than once or not at all.

Questions:

1 A 38-year-old woman presents to the A & E with generalised tonic-clonic convulsions. She becomes unconscious. An ultrasound report is found in her medical record, which shows a live 10-week intrauterine pregnancy.

2 A 23-year-old primigravida is noted to have a BP of 150/90 mmHg at a routine antenatal visit. She recollects mild intermittent headaches but is otherwise asymptomatic. She is now 18 weeks pregnant and has no proteinuria.

3 A 30-year-old second gravida records a BP of 160/110 mmHG when she attends the day assessment unit for her fetal monitoring. She is now 30 weeks into her pregnancy with monochorionic monoamniotic twin gestation with no major complications. Her urinalysis shows 4+ proteinuria. Further analysis shows serum uric acid of 6.8 mg/dL and a normal complete blood count with mild elevation of liver enzymes. An intravenous access is obtained immediately, blood investigations are sent, the bladder is catheterised and she is shifted to the high dependency unit.

4 A 30-year-old primigravida is admitted in spontaneous labour at 37 weeks gestation. Her antenatal period was uneventful. Her BP reading is 140/90 mmHG with 1+ proteinuria. She is now having regular uterine contractions and vaginal examination revealed a 3 cm dilated cervix.

For answers, see 2.14.

1.15 Induction of labour

Options:

A   amniotomy
B   amniotomy followed by oxytocin infusion
C   category III LSCS
D   cervical stretch and sweep of membranes
E   counselling
F   extra-amniotic PGE2 gel
G   intracervical Foley balloon
H   intracervical prostaglandin E2 gel
I   oral misoprostol 25 mcg
J   oxytocin infusion with continuous fetal heart monitoring
K   bowel prep enema
L   prostaglandin F2 alpha
M   vaginal misoprostol 25 mcg
N   vaginal prostaglandin E2 gel

For each of the following questions, choose the *single*-most appropriate intervention from the list A–N. Each option may be chosen once, more than once or not at all.

Questions:

1   A 23-year-old primigravida at 38 weeks gestation complains of reduced fetal movements for the past 2 days. Her antenatal course was uneventful and her current observations are within normal limits. Further evaluation shows normal estimated fetal weight on ultrasound with marked oligohydramnios and normal UA and MCA Doppler study. She denies any vaginal discharge. Vaginal examination shows a Bishop score of 5 and membrane sweep has been done.

2   A 23-year-old woman with two previous normal deliveries attends the antenatal clinic at 37 weeks gestation with backache. Her current pregnancy is a dichorionic diamniotic twin gestation with no comorbidities. Both fetuses show normal growth pattern in cephalic presentation. Her Bishop score is 5. An elective induction is due at 38 weeks gestation.

3   A 29-year-old primigravida is being reviewed at term +10 in the consultant antenatal clinic. Her BMI is 28. She perceives movements well and admission CTG is normal. Vaginal examination shows a Bishop score of 3 and has had a stretch and sweep by her midwife.

4   A 24-year-old woman who is a third gravida attends the antenatal clinic with her third-trimester ultrasound report at 37 weeks gestation requesting delivery by Caesarean section. Her previous two pregnancies were spontaneous miscarriages at 8 and 10 week gestations, respectively. She underwent surgical terminations and had received anti-D both times. Her indirect Coombs test has been negative. She is noted to have polyhydramnios with an AFI of 20. Fetal umbilical and middle cerebral artery Doppler study is within normal limits. No other obvious anomalies were noted.

For answers, see 2.15.

1.16 Management of labour

Options:

A amniotomy
B Caesarean section
C continuous fetal heart monitoring and expectant management
D enema
E fetal scalp blood pH
F fetal scalp electrode
G intermittent fetal heart monitoring
H intracervical Foley's balloon
I intracervical prostaglandin E2 gel
J oral misoprostol 25 mcg
K oxytocin infusion with continuous fetal heart monitoring
L prostaglandin F2 alpha
M vaginal misoprostol 25 mcg
N vaginal prostaglandin E2 gel

For each of the following questions, choose the *single*-most appropriate option from the list A–N. Each option may be chosen once, more than once or not at all.

Questions:

1 A 30-year-old primigravida comes to the delivery suite with regular uterine contractions and leaking vaginal for 4 hours. She has completed 39 weeks gestation, with an uneventful antenatal period. She perceives fetal movements well. On examination, it was found that her uterus is contracting well and vaginal examination reveals a 4 cm dilated, well-effaced cervix, with vertex at –3 station. Clear liquor is noted.

2 A 28-year-old third gravida is admitted in spontaneous labour at term +4 gestation. Her previous deliveries were normal at term. She is progressing well and is being monitored by regular, intermittent auscultation. She was noted to be 4 cm dilated and an amniotomy was done. Clear liquor was seen. Four hours after amniotomy, vaginal examination is repeated as the uterine contractions are 4–5 in 10 minutes with stronger intensity. Cervical lips are found to be very thick and edematous with 6 cm dilatation. Vertex is at –3 station with marked caput and moulding formation.

3 A primigravida is being induced for oligohydramnios and reduced fetal movements at 39 weeks gestation. She is known to have an 8 cm fibroid near the fundus. Serial growth scans are within normal limits. Oxytocin infusion is commenced and continuous fetal heart monitoring is reassuring. She was noted to be 4 cm dilated and an amniotomy was performed. Four hours later repeat examination shows cervix to be 6 cm dilated, with minimal clear liquor draining.

4   A 30-year-old third gravida with dichorionic diamniotic twin pregnancy at 37 week of gestation has spontaneous onset of labour. Fifteen minutes after the first twin delivery, uterus is found to be relaxed, with fetal head in the pelvis at –2 station. Fetal heart rate is 146 bpm with good variability.

For answers, see 2.16.

1.17 Multiple pregnancy

Options:

A amniocentesis
B bed rest and protein supplement
C betamethasone 12 mg, two doses 12 hours apart
D consultant-led antenatal care in fetal medicine unit
E elective lower segment Caesarean section
F emergency lower segment Caesarean section
G fetal Doppler study
H fetal echocardiogram
I in patient care and steroids (betamethasone 12 mg two doses)
J induction of labour with prostaglandins
K iron and nutritional supplement
L prophylactic cervical cerclage
M reassurance
N selective termination
O serial growth scans 2–3 weekly
P oxytocin infusion with twin monitoring

For each of the following questions, choose the *single*-most appropriate management option from the list A–N. Each option may be chosen once, more than once or not at all.

Questions:

1 A 26-year-old primigravida with MCDA twin gestation attends the antenatal clinic with her 20-week anomaly scan report. Both twins are structurally normal with no other abnormality.

2 A 30-year-old second gravida with DCDA twin gestation presents at 32 weeks gestation with mild abdominal discomfort. Her first delivery was an emergency Caesarean section for failed induction. She denies any bleeding or draining. On examination, her uterus is found to be soft, non-tender and overdistended. Fetal hearts rates of both twins are normal. Irregular tightening is noted. Vaginal examination reveals multiparous cervix with no dilatation and presenting part above the brim.

3 A 28-year-old primigravida with dichorionic diamniotic twin gestation attends the antenatal clinic with her third-trimester growth scan report at 28 weeks gestation. She had been started on aspirin earlier in the pregnancy. Twin A is in cephalic presentation and twin B is in transverse position. All fetal parameters are less than the 10th centile with normal liquor and normal Doppler study.

4 A 30-year-old woman has been diagnosed with triplet gestation at 8 weeks gestation. She was offered counselling and advised selective termination, which she declined. She is now 13 weeks pregnant with normal nuchal translucency scan in all the three fetuses.

For answers, see 2.17.

1.18 Assisted vaginal delivery

Options:

A abandon vaginal delivery and proceed with Cat 1 LSCS
B category 1 LSCS under general anaesthesia
C category II LSCS
D catheterisation and expectant management
E epidural anaesthesia and continuous fetal heart monitoring
F episiotomy and pudendal block
G expectant management with continuous fetal heart monitoring
H fetal scalp electrode and monitoring
I Kielland rotational forceps
J low or mid-cavity forceps
K manual rotation followed by forceps delivery
L outlet forceps
M rotation with vacuum cup followed by delivery
N trial vaginal delivery in operating theatre
O ventouse delivery with Kiwi cup

For each of the following questions, choose the *single*-most appropriate intervention from the list A–O. Each option may be chosen once, more than once or not at all.

Questions:

1 A 28-year-old primigravida is being induced for gestational diabetes. She is now at 38 weeks gestation and is on insulin therapy. Her recent blood sugars and HbA1c were high. She has had vaginal prostaglandin E2 gel instilled the previous night. The following morning, her cervix is found to be 0.5 cm long and 2 cm dilated. Oxytocin infusion is started after amniotomy with continuous fetal heart monitoring. Four hours later, vaginal examination reveals a 4-cm dilated cervix. Four hours later, she is found to have a fully dilated cervix with vertex presentation at –2 station. She is encouraged to push and 2 hours later vertex is at +2 station with a small caput and fetal heart rate is reassuring.

2 A 29-year-old lady presents with PPROM at 34 weeks gestation to the delivery suite. She is not in active labour and receives a course of steroids and erythromycin. She presents 2 days later feeling unwell. Her abdomen shows a soft non-tender uterus with reassuring fetal heart. Labour is induced in view of raised CRP. At 4 pm her cervix is found to be 4 cm dilated with absent membranes. Four hours later, the cervix is found to be fully dilated and she is encouraged to bear down with the contractions. Two hours later, fetal heart monitoring reveals late decelerations and the vertex is at +2 station with LOA position.

3   A 30-year-old primigravida is admitted in spontaneous labour at term. She has good uterine contractions. The partogram reveals cervical dilatation at 12 noon to be 4 cm and at 4 pm it is 5 cm. Oxytocin infusion is started. At 8 pm she is found to be fully dilated, when she is encouraged to push. At 10 pm vertex is found to be at +1 station with ROT position. Manual rotation is attempted twice followed by rotation with kiwi cup under pudendal block but is unsuccessful. Position is still ROT.

4   A 29-year-old primigravida is admitted in spontaneous labour at 39 weeks gestation. She is known to have idiopathic thrombocytopenic purpura and is on steroids. Her current blood reports are normal. She is noted to be fully dilated with vertex at 0 station 4 hours after admission. Amniotomy is done and she is encouraged to push. Vertex is in LOA at pelvic floor level. Fetal heart shows late decelerations.

For answers, see 2.18.

1.19 Intrauterine fetal demise

Options:

A   artificial rupture of membranes
B   emergency lower segment Caesarean section
C   commence intravenous antibiotics with anaerobic cover
D   counselling
E   expectant management and referral to higher centre
F   extra amniotic catheter insertion
G   HDU admission, correction of hypoglycaemia, coagulation and electrolytes
H   intracervical Foley balloon
I   Kleihauer test and anti-D administration
J   mifepristone followed by vaginal misoprostol
K   oral misoprostol 25 mcg
L   oxytocin infusion 5 units in 500 mL of normal saline
M   ursodeoxycholic acid 300 mg twice daily
N   vaginal prostaglandin E2 gel
O   vitamin K injection and fresh frozen plasma

For each of the following questions, choose the *single*-most appropriate intervention from the list A–N. Each option may be chosen once, more than once or not at all.

Questions:

1   A 24-year-old woman in her second pregnancy was referred from the radiology department following an ultrasound at 24 weeks gestation. She was diagnosed with monochorionic diamniotic twin gestation earlier. Her ultrasound study today showed fetal demise of one twin and a well-grown second twin. Counselling has been offered and initial blood tests have been sent.

2   A 28-year-old woman presents to the antenatal clinic at 32 weeks gestation with loss of fetal movements for the past 2 days. Her antenatal period was uneventful except fetal bilateral pelviectasis at 20-week anomaly scan, which was reported to be normal on a subsequent ultrasound scan. Clinical examination is normal, but an obstetric ultrasound reveals fetal demise.

3   An 18-year-old primigravida attends the day assessment unit at 36 weeks gestation with loss of fetal movements. She was diagnosed with obstetric cholestasis and was started on ursodeoxycholic acid 3 weeks ago. Ultrasound confirms intrauterine fetal demise. She and her partner are counselled and initial blood tests are done. She opts for immediate obstetric management.

4   A 27-year-old woman presents with abdominal cramps and vaginal bleeding at term +2 days in her second pregnancy. Her blood group is rhesus negative and was given anti-D after her first delivery. Further tests confirm placental abruption and fetal

demise. She looks pale with a PR of 100 bpm, and her BP is 100/60 mmHG. Her Bishop score is 3. Immediate intravenous access is obtained and blood tests are sent.

5   A 30-year-old primigravida presents with loss of fetal movements for the past 2 days at 30 weeks gestation. She also recollects having dark urine for the past 2 weeks. On examination she is found to be icteric, dehydrated and tachycardic. Ultrasound examination, confirms fetal demise and blood analysis shows severely deranged liver enzymes with INR of 3.0. Vaginal examination shows a very unfavourable cervix.

For answers, see 2.19.

1.20 Psychiatric disease in pregnancy and puerperium

Options:

A   advice against breastfeeding
B   advice against pregnancy
C   advice on diet exercise and folic acid
D   antipsychotic drugs
E   cognitive behavioural therapy (CBT)
F   counselling
G   counselling the partner and other family members
H   dedicated mother and baby unit admission
I   electroconvulsive therapy
J   interpersonal psychotherapy IPT
K   involve social services
L   involvement of special mental health team/psychiatrist
M   rapid tranquillisation
N   SSRI – fluoxetine
O   tricyclic antidepressants – imipramine

For each of the following questions, choose the *single*-most appropriate option from the list A–O. Each option may be chosen once, more than once or not at all.

Questions:

1   A 21-year-old woman with known bipolar disorder on regular medication attends for preconception counselling. She is on fluoxetine and is on regular follow-up.

2   A 30-year-old woman presents to the delivery suite at 32 weeks gestation with severe backache. She denies any vaginal watery loss or bleeding. On examination, her vital signs are found to be stable, with a soft uterus. Vaginal examination was not performed as she does not consent. Her recent growth scan has been normal. On further questioning, she lacks coherence and says she heard voices the night before, which instructed her to go to the hospital immediately.

3   A 22-year-old primigravida attends the breastfeeding clinic on the 7th day following her delivery. She is tearful due to her inability to feed the baby and feels completely worthless. She lives alone and says life means nothing to her now and talks about harming herself. She looks emaciated and dehydrated.

4   A 34-year-old woman attends the postnatal clinic feeling tired with lack of appetite and feeling unwell on the 4th day following her delivery. She is complaining of severe pain in the episiotomy site and vaginal bleeding. She had a prolonged labour following induction and a forceps delivery. She is very upset about the whole event. Physical examination reveals normal findings and stable vital parameters.

5   A 29-year-old woman is attending the GP surgery for breast engorgement. She was a victim of road traffic accident recently and lost her baby at term due to placental abruption. She was induced and had vaginal delivery and discharged later from the hospital. She was prescribed cabergoline following the delivery. On examination, there is very mild breast tenderness with no engorgement and is extremely tearful.

For answers, see 2.20.

1.21 Surgical problems/abdominal pain in pregnancy

Options:

A   acute appendicitis
B   acute cholecystitis
C   acute pancreatitis
D   acute severe gastritis
E   constipation with faecal impaction
F   hydronephrosis
G   incarceration of uterus with urinary retention
H   Meckel's diverticulitis
I   placental abruption
J   preterm labour
K   red degeneration of fibroid
L   severe hyperemesis
M   sickle cell crisis
N   ulcerative colitis
O   urinary tract sepsis

For each of the following questions, choose the *single*-most appropriate diagnosis from the list A–O. Each option may be chosen once, more than once or not at all.

Questions:

1   A 22-year-old woman presents with severe abdominal pain to accident and emergency at 12-week gestation. She denies any bleeding or urinary symptoms but has severe nausea. The night before she had been to a party and had consumed alcohol. Her BP is 110/80 mmHG, PR 98 bpm and abdominal examination reveals diffuse tenderness over her upper abdomen with no rigidity or guarding. She had undergone routine nuchal translucency ultrasound the day before.

2   A 30-year-old third gravid lady presents to the delivery suite with abdominal discomfort and difficulty in passing urine since afternoon. She is 14 weeks pregnant and her NT scan had been normal a week ago. Her BP is 120/80 mmHG, PR 88 bpm and an abdominal examination reveals fullness in lower abdomen with no rigidity or guarding.

3   A 20-year-old primigravida presents to accident and emergency department at 18-week gestation with severe abdominal pain and vomiting. She denies any vaginal bleeding or urinary symptoms. She is febrile, with a BP of 130/80 mmHG, PR 109 bpm and white cell count 20,000/μL. Abdominal examination reveals right-sided abdominal tenderness, guarding and rigidity. On palpation, the uterus is soft, with normal fetal heart.

4   A 24-year-old primigravida presents at 28 weeks gestation with dull ache over the abdomen, radiating towards the back since the past few weeks. She has dysuria, flank pain, frequent urination and intermittent fever for which she had received antibiotics 4 weeks earlier. On examination, she is found to be febrile, with BP 100/80 mmHg and PR 78 bpm.

Abdominal examination reveals a soft non-tender uterus, with tenderness in the lumbar region. Vaginal examination is unremarkable.

5   A 32-year-old primigravida presents at 30 weeks gestation with severe abdominal pain. She is known to have fibroids and was given a course of steroids the previous week, as she presented with a similar episode. On examination, she is found to be dehydrated with a PR of 110 bpm, BP of 120/70 mmHG and tenderness over the uterus, with no cervical changes. She denies any bleeding and ultrasound examination shows appropriate fetal growth and no placental pathology.

For answers, see 2.21.

1.22 Impaired glucose metabolism in pregnancy

Options:

A   commence insulin sliding scale regimen
B   commence oral metformin
C   fasting and postprandial sugar, HbA1c level monitoring
D   folic acid, diet and exercises along with monitoring
E   home glucose monitoring
F   induction of labour at 37 completed weeks
G   induction of labour at 40 weeks
H   insulin treatment
I   low-dose (75 mg) aspirin
J   lower segment Caesarean section
K   offer induction of labour
L   OGTT (oral glucose tolerance test)
M   renal and retinal screening
N   thromboprophylaxis with enoxaparin 40 mg

For each of the following questions, choose the *single*-most appropriate option from the list A–N. Each option may be chosen once, more than once or not at all.

Questions:

1   A 28-year-old primigravida attends the combined diabetes antenatal clinic for consultant-led care at 8-week gestation. She has type 1 diabetes and is on insulin. Her BMI is 28. Her most recent blood profile is as follows: fasting plasma glucose level of 6 mmol/L and HbA1c level is 6.0% (43 mmol/mol). She monitors her glucose levels and undergoes annual retinal screening

2   A 34-year-old primigravida is seen in the antenatal clinic at 32 weeks gestation. Her BMI is 28. Her growth scan showed polyhydramnios. Her 20-week anatomy scan was normal. Her oral OGTT (fasting) with 75 g of glucose is 7.8 mmol/L, HbA1c 8.0% (64 mmol/mol). Her renal parameters are normal.

3   A 39-year-old second gravida is being reviewed after her third-trimester growth scan at 37 completed weeks. During her first pregnancy, she had fetal demise at 29 weeks gestation and labour was induced. She has type 2 diabetes and is on insulin and metformin 750 mg twice daily. Her BMI is 30. Her most recent blood profile is as follows: fasting glucose 6.2 mmol/L, HbA1c 6.5% (48 mmol/mol). The ultrasound is within normal limits and the AC measures above the 97th centile.

4   A 30-year-old second gravid woman attends the antenatal clinic with a nuchal translucency report at 13 weeks gestation. She developed gestational diabetes in her previous pregnancy and was on metformin. She had an emergency Caesarean section at 39 weeks for failed induction. Her sugar levels were completely normal 6 weeks post-delivery.

For answers, see 2.22.

1.23 Antepartum haemorrhage

Options:

A   amniotomy
B   betamethasone 12 mg two doses at 24 hours interval
C   cardiopulmonary resuscitation
D   category I LSCS
E   conservative treatment
F   continuous fetal heart monitoring
G   fresh frozen plasma
H   indirect Coombs test
I   initial resuscitation followed by category I LSCS
J   inpatient care
K   IV access, CBC, coagulation profile, liver function test, urea and electrolytes, cross-match 6 units of blood
L   Kleihauer test and anti-D 300 mcg administration
M   obstetric ultrasound
N   reassurance

For each of the following questions, choose the *single*-most appropriate option from the list A–N. Each option may be chosen once, more than once or not at all.

Questions:

1   A 34-year-old woman presents to the delivery suite at 36 weeks gestation with contractions and vaginal bleeding. Her previous two pregnancies were mid-trimester miscarriages and currently she has had a cervical cerclage done at 14 weeks gestation. On examination, she is found to be contracting twice in 10 minutes, with uterus relaxing in between. Her vitals are normal. Vaginal examination reveals a well-effaced thin cervix, 3 cm dilated with mild bleeding. Cervical suture is removed. CTG is normal.

2   A 23-year-old primigravida attends the delivery suite at 30 weeks with vaginal bleeding and abdominal pain since 2 two hours. She looks pale with a PR of 110 bpm and BP of 100/60 mmHg. She finds the examination painful. Fetal heart rate is 98 bpm with a suspicious CTG. Vaginal examination reveals an uneffaced cervix with bleeding.

3   A 28-year-old primigravida attends the day assessment unit at 39 weeks gestation with abdominal pain and vaginal bleeding since an hour. Her antenatal period was uneventful. On examination, it was found that she has regular uterine contractions with a reassuring fetal heart trace. Vaginal examination reveals a well-effaced 4 cm dilated cervix with mild bloodstained discharge.

4   A 29-year-old second gravida presents at 30-week gestation with a small vaginal bleed. She denies any abdominal pain. She is haemodynamically stable. Abdominal examination reveals a soft non-tender uterus. Fetal heart trace is reassuring. She delivered her first baby by LSCS at 34 weeks gestation following spontaneous rupture of membranes with breech presentation.

For answers, see 2.23.

1.24 Respiratory diseases in pregnancy

Options:

A anti-tuberculosis treatment
B beta-agonists and regular Montelukast
C complete blood count, urea, creatinine, LFT and peripheral smear
D counselling
E CT pulmonary angiogram
F high dependency care with high flow oxygen, antibiotics and hydration
G immediate nebulisation, beta-agonist and steroid inhalers and start Montelukast
H immediate resuscitation with CPAP
I inpatient care with hydration, antibiotics and physiotherapy
J inpatient care for monitoring
K nutritional supplements with iron and folic acid
L oral azithromycin 500 mg once daily
M pulmonary function tests
N reassurance
O systemic steroids

For each of the following questions, choose the *single*-most appropriate management option from the list A–N. Each option may be chosen once, more than once or not at all.

Questions:

1   A 27-year-old primigravida attends the accident and emergency department at 20 weeks gestation with severe breathlessness. Her BMI is 24. She denies any chest tightness or pain. She is known to have hyperactive airway syndrome and was on Montelukast, which she had stopped earlier when her pregnancy was confirmed. She is afebrile with PR of 100 bpm, BP of 100/60 mmHG, respiratory rate 40 bpm and SaO$_2$ 94% and PEFR 35%. Chest auscultation shows poor air entry on both sides.

2   A 35-year-old third gravida attends the delivery suite at 20 weeks gestation with difficulty in breathing, right-sided chest pain and palpitations. She booked late at 16 weeks in this pregnancy. She was a chronic smoker but quit a few years ago. Her BMI is 32. She had undergone cardiac evaluation prior to this pregnancy with normal. She is on regular steroids and beta-agonist inhalers. On examination, her PR is 90 bpm, respiratory rate 30/minute and PEFR >70%. ECG shows sinus tachycardia. She is admitted in the HDU and is clinically stable.

3   A 17-year-old primigravida presents to the day assessment unit at 28 weeks gestation for breathlessness on exertion. She denies smoking. Her BMI is 20. She looks pale with a PR of 78 bpm, BP 100/60 mmHG and SaO$_2$ 98%. There are no uterine contractions and her CTG is normal. Her haemoglobin is 9.0 g with MCV of 65 fL. Her ECG shows normal sinus rhythm.

4 A 20-year-old second gravida attends the day assessment unit with fever, cough and breathlessness at 28 weeks gestation. She is a non-smoker with a BMI of 22. On examination, she is found to be febrile, dehydrated with a respiratory rate of 30/minute and PR of 103 bpm, with crepitations heard on both sides of her lung fields. She brings up copious purulent sputum.

For answers, see 2.24.

1.25 Risk management in obstetrics

Options:

A   auditing the existing practice and outcome
B   call for help
C   counselling
D   discussion with clinical lead
E   evidence-based practice
F   immediate reporting to police
G   immediate resuscitation and transfer to high dependency unit
H   incident reporting
I   initiate disciplinary action against the person involved
J   initiate root cause analysis
K   initiate serious untoward incident investigation (SUI)
L   multidisciplinary meeting
M   revise and formulate new protocol
N   revise the existing guidelines and disseminating to all antenatal staff
O   seek trust lawyer's advice

For each of the following questions, choose the *single*-most appropriate management option from the list A–O. Each option may be chosen once, more than once or not at all.

Questions:

1   A 26-year-old primigravida attends the day assessment unit at term +2 for loss of fetal movements. Subsequent ultrasound examination confirms intrauterine fetal demise. Her antenatal course was normal and her third-trimester growth scan showed an adequately grown fetus with normal liquor. She has attended the day assessment unit a few days ago with the same complaint when cardiotocograph was found to be normal. She was reassured and advised to return to hospital if any further problems occurred. She and her partner are informed about the fetal demise and counselled by the team. She is very upset and opts for induction of labour the next day.

2   A 32-year-old second gravida has a spontaneous delivery in a district hospital. Uterine atony is encountered. As part of resuscitation, a team member was asked to arrange blood cross-matching and a sample error occurs. The wrong blood bag has been dispatched. At the beginning of transfusion, the patient develops severe reactions and the problem is recognised immediately.

3   A 19-year-old girl was admitted in early labour at term. She had not returned to the antenatal clinic after her anomaly scan at 20 weeks gestation. She does not speak English and examination showed severe external genital synechia. She progresses quickly and delivers a 6-pound (2722 g) baby. Further examination reveals a fourth-degree tear, which gets recognised and dealt by a senior obstetricians. Incident reporting was done. She undergoes repair in theatre.

4   A 28-year-old woman reports to the delivery suite at 32 weeks gestation with painless vaginal bleeding. Her first baby was born at term by Caesarean section. Placenta accreta was suspected by earlier ultrasound examination and further MRI confirms accreta. She was offered counselling and advised inpatient care. She undergoes an emergency Caesarean section and hysterectomy for complete placenta accreta.

For answers, see 2.25.

1.26 Intrauterine growth restriction

Options:

A   amniocentesis
B   amniotic fluid assessment
C   bed rest and nutritional support
D   betamethasone 12 mg two doses
E   biophysical profile assessment biweekly
F   category 2 lower segment Caesarean section
G   category 3 lower segment Caesarean section
H   commence low-dose aspirin
I   cytomegalovirus and toxoplasmosis screening
J   induction of labour with intravaginal prostaglandins
K   reassurance
L   screening for Zika virus infection
M   serial growth scans, fetal umbilical Doppler study
N   sildenafil
O   uterine artery Doppler

For each of the following questions, choose the *single*-most appropriate intervention from the list A–N. Each option may be chosen once, more than once or not at all.

Questions:

1   A 27-year-old second gravida is referred by her midwife for small dates on palpation at 28 weeks gestation. Her BMI is 18. Her first trimester serum screening was negative. In her first pregnancy, she delivered a 4.8-pound (2177 g) baby at term. Ultrasound shows all fetal parameters less than 5th centile with normal Doppler indices.

2   A 19-year-old primigravida with a BMI of 30 reports after her first trimester serum screening and NT scan, which shows low PAPP–A.

3   A 28-year-old second gravida attends the antenatal clinic after her anomaly scan at 20 weeks, which shows symmetrical IUGR and normal fetal anatomy. The fetal bowel appears echogenic uterine artery Doppler is normal. She has not had any antenatal visits earlier in the current pregnancy. Her first pregnancy ended with spontaneous miscarriage at 16 weeks gestation.

4   A 34-year-old primigravida presents at 35 weeks gestation with reduced perception of fetal movements. She is a non-smoker with a BMI of 27 and clinically small for dates baby. Ultrasound reports fetal biometry uniformly less than the 2nd percentile, amniotic fluid index of 6, and umbilical artery Doppler shows a reversed end diastolic flow.

For answers, see 2.26.

1.27 Haematological diseases in pregnancy

Options:

A   acute myeloid leukemia
B   alpha thalassemia
C   aplastic anaemia
D   disseminated intravascular coagulation
E   drug-induced anaemia
F   drug-induced thrombocytopenia
G   HELLP syndrome
H   hereditary spherocytosis
I   idiopathic thrombocytopenic purpura
J   iron deficiency anaemia
K   megaloblastic anaemia
L   nutritional anaemia
M   sickle cell crisis
N   systemic lupus erythematosus

For each of the following questions, choose the *single*-most appropriate diagnosis from the list A–N. Each option may be chosen once, more than once or not at all.

Questions:

1   An 18-year-old primigravida presents at 20 weeks gestation with extreme lethargy and tiredness to the delivery suite. She smokes 10 cigarettes a day and lives alone. She has not been to the doctors or midwives after her booking. Her current blood results are Hb – 9.0 g/dL; MCV – 70 fL; haematocrit – 35%; serum ferritin – 45 mcg/L (ng/mL); total count – 11×10^9/L; platelets – 375×10^9/L.

2   A 23-year-old primigravida is being reviewed with her blood results at 12 weeks gestation. Her blood results are as follows: full blood count Hb – 5.0 g/dL; MCV – 90 fL; total count – 1×10^9/L; platelets – 80×10^9/L. She admits feeling lethargic and complains of generalised weakness. On examination, she is found to be pale with a few petechial spots, which she attributes to a recent viral illness. On repeating the blood tests, almost similar results are revealed.

3   A 20-year-old primigravida presents at 12 weeks gestation with gum bleeding to the general practitioner, who then arranges a full blood count. The results are as follows: full blood count Hb – 11.0 g/dL; MCV – 90 fL; total count – 8×10^9/L; platelets – 100×10^9/L. Repeat examination reveals a platelet count of 80×10^9/L. She suffers from menorrhagia and gum bleeding since many years.

4   A 26-year-old Asian woman presents to the day assessment unit with swelling in her legs, headache and feeling unwell at 32-week gestation. On examination, her BP is found to be 160/110 mmHG and PR 88 bpm. Urine analysis shows 3+ of protein. Full blood count results are as follows: Hb – 10.0 g/dL; MCV – 90 fL; total count – 11 × 10⁹/L; platelets – 50 × 10⁹/L.

For answers, see 2.27.

Chapter 2: Obstetric Answers

2.1 Preconception counselling

1   **G**

High-dose folic acid is needed in view of obesity.
(See further: *CMACE/RCOG Joint Guideline: Management of Women with Obesity in Pregnancy*)

2   **J**

Single functioning kidney is not a high-risk factor in an otherwise healthy woman. Routine use of periconceptional folic acid is adequate.

3   **A**

Pulmonary hypertension worsens in pregnancy. Moderate and severe pulmonary hypertension is likely to worsen and even be fatal in some patients. (See further: *CEMACH Saving Mothers' Lives: Pulmonary Hypertension, Marfan's with Aortic Involvement, and Significant Aortic Stenosis or Ventricular Dysfunction 5%–30% Mortality*)

4   **M**

Routine rubella immunity status should be checked other than advice to quit smoking and commence folic acid.

5   **M**

As she is currently well and contemplating pregnancy, she should be supported in her choices. Routine rubella status and folate is recommended. (See further: *Antenatal and Postnatal Mental Health: Clinical Management and Service Guidance. Clinical Guideline [CG192]*. Published: December 2014; updated: August 2017)

2.2 Management of early pregnancy

1 G

An urgent ultrasound examination is required to image the pregnancy as an ectopic pregnancy must be ruled out before an acute urinary sepsis.

2 C

Catheterisation to relieve the acute urinary retention. It is common with a retroverted uterus in the early weeks of gestation.

3 M

No further intervention is needed in a threatened miscarriage.

4 H

Laparoscopic salpingectomy and allowing the intrauterine pregnancy to continue will be the next step in management.

5 J

Selective reduction and counselling about options and outcomes is essential.

2.3 Infections in pregnancy

1   E

Acute urinary sepsis is still an important reason for admission to the intensive care unit. Careful attention must be paid to avoid deterioration.

2   J

Herpes viral infection leads to acute pain and urinary symptoms.
(See further: *Management of Genital Herpes in Pregnancy: Joint Guideline with the British Association for Sexual Health and HIV (BASHH) and RCOG.* 2014)

3   K

Oral aciclovir should be prescribed for pregnant women with chickenpox if they present within 24 hours of the onset of the rash and if they are 20 + 0 weeks of gestation or beyond.
(See further: *Chickenpox in Pregnancy. Green-top Guideline No. 13*)

4   B

Caesarean section is recommended for all women presenting with primary episode genital herpes lesions at the time of delivery in order to reduce exposure of the fetus to HSV which may be present in maternal genital secretion.

5   D

First dose of hepatitis B vaccine and one dose of hepatitis B immune globulin (HBIG) should be offered to newborn within 24 hours of birth.

2.4 Antenatal screening I

1   C

Chorionic villus sampling and genetic testing should be offered to the couple.

2   A

If both parents are cystic fibrosis carriers, the fetus has one in four chance of having cystic fibrosis. Amniocentesis and genetic testing should be offered.

3   I

If one partner is a carrier, there is one in four chance of the baby being a carrier. If both are found to be carriers, there is a one in four chance of the fetus being affected by thalassemia major.

4   G

Duchenne muscular dystrophy is inherited in an X-linked recessive pattern. Each son born to a carrier female has a 50% chance of inheriting the DBMD mutation and having MD. Each daughter born to a carrier female instead has a 50% chance of inheriting the DBMD mutation and becoming a carrier like her mother.

2.5 Antenatal screening II

1   J

Choroid plexus cyst is a common soft marker noted in 0.2%–3% of all pregnancies. It is associated with trisomy 18.

2   M

Short femur in the absence of other deformities is usually constitutional. It could represent intrauterine growth restriction.

3   C

CVS is indicated as the risk of aneuploidy is high.

4   I

Isolated renal pelviectasis needs postnatal follow-up of ultrasound scans.

2.6 Preterm labour/PPROM

1   M

Oral erythromycin for 10 days along with steroids should be considered.
(See further: *Preterm Pre-labour Rupture of Membranes. Green-top Guideline No. 44*. Published: November 2006; updated: October 2010)

2   A

Steroid for fetal lung maturity is the priority in this situation.

3   B

Emergency LSCS is warranted.

4   E

Insertion of rescue cerclage has a role in this situation.
(See further: *Cervical Cerclage. Green-top Guideline No. 60*. May 2011)

5   B

Placental abruption is the clinical diagnosis.

2.7 Post-partum haemorrhage I

1   O

Immediate resuscitation is the priority in the management of any obstetric emergency.

2   C

B-Lynch sutures should be considered after initial pharmacological agents.
(See further: *Green-top Guideline No. 52.* May 2009; Minor revisions November 2009 and April 2011)

3   E

Continuous bladder drainage with a Foley catheter and continuous monitoring is required after the initial management.

4   D

Analgesia and good lighting are very important for adequate perineal repair.

5   P

Pharmacological (uterotonic) agents are the first-line treatment of PPH.

2.8 Post-partum haemorrhage II

1 **K**

Early decision for hysterectomy is indicated with adequate counselling debriefing. (See further: *Placenta Praevia, Accreta and Vasa Praevia: Diagnosis and Management. Green-top Guideline No. 27.* January 2011)

2 **P**

Intravenous access and arranging blood or blood products is important in initial management of PPH.

3 **H**

Carboprost is the next drug of choice as ergot alkaloids are contraindicated.

2.9 Acute intrapartum events

1   O

Prevention of cord compression by physical methods while arrangements are being made for Caesarean section. Umbilical cord prolapse is the diagnosis.
(See further: *Green-top Guideline No. 50*. November 2014)

2   A

Call for help is the first response in shoulder dystocia. Acronym HELLPER

3   A

Water birth is encouraged for low-risk women in labour and hence the availability of senior staff nearby is unlikely. After calling for help follow ABCD of resuscitation.

4   C

Uterine rupture needs to be considered and decision delivery interval needs to be as early as possible.

5   L

ABC – MOET guidelines.

2.10 Maternal collapse I

1   **M**

Basic resuscitation airway, breathing and circulation.

2   **E**

High dependency unit admission, stabilisation and further evaluation is the standard protocol in managing a stable but sick patient. Meningitis with post-operative abdominal pain is likely.

3   **E**

Probable diagnosis is diabetic ketoacidosis.

4   **F**

Category I Caesarean section is indicated as the mother is stable but the fetus is in severe distress due to placental abruption.

5   **A**

As this patient is already in a hospital environment, coordinating further help is the priority.

2.11 Maternal collapse II

1 F

Substance misuse and related metabolic sequences need to be ruled out.

2 C

Coronary angiogram and the cardiologist need to be involved as part of multidisciplinary management.

3 L

Cerebrovascular event needs to be excluded.

4 A

It may be an anxiety-related panic attack or pain shock or a more sinister cause. Basic resuscitative measures need to be initiated first.

2.12 Domestic violence

1   C

Offering confidential counselling to the teen pregnant woman is the first step towards management. It may be a covert plea for help with difficult personal or social circumstances.

2   K

In addition to the medical treatment, liaising with social services for further follow-up is vital as most of the time medical professionals are the only people these patients present themselves to. She is 15 years old and is a minor.

3   A

Establishing a good rapport with the patient is an important first step in managing any pregnant woman. It is better to avoid the family for translation purposes.

4   N

Screening for other STIs, contact tracing, treatment and counselling is done by qualified health care professionals in GUM clinics.

5   J

Further management needs to be discussed with the patient and the decision for Caesarean section made if necessary.

6   K

Domestic abuse should be kept in mind in these situations and social services help needs to be sought.
(See further: *Domestic Violence and Abuse: Multi-agency Working. NICE Guidelines [PH50]*. Published: February 2014)

2.13 Thromboembolism in pregnancy

1   C

After initial resuscitation, treatment dose of enoxaparin needs to be commenced. Computerised tomographic pulmonary angiogram is done to diagnose pulmonary embolism as the next step.

2   C

Therapeutic dose of low molecular weight heparin should be commenced. (See further: *Thromboembolic Disease in Pregnancy and the Puerperium: Acute Management. Green-top Guideline No. 37b. April 2015*)

3   B

Women with thrombophilia should receive 50%–60% of therapeutic dose of LMWH (See further: *Reducing the Risk of Venous Thromboembolism during Pregnancy and the Puerperium. Green-top Guideline No. 37a. April 2015*)

4   N

Post-delivery thromboprophylaxis with enoxaparin is recommended.

5   A

Inferior vena cava filters need to be considered in women with recurrent embolism to prevent pulmonary embolism.

2.14 Hypertensive disorders in pregnancy

1   **B**

Immediate resuscitation is the priority.

2   **G**

Oral labetalol is the drug of choice.

3   **L**

Prevention of seizures is the next step in management, and magnesium sulfate is the drug of choice.

4   **D**

Baseline blood parameters and continuous monitoring is essential as one-third of these patients have later.

2.15 Induction of labour

1   N

Vaginal prostaglandins E2 gel is the choice of induction.

2   D

Membrane sweeping is offered prior to pharmacological induction.

3   N

Vaginal prostaglandin E2 gel is the choice of induction.

4   E

Good counselling regarding induction of labour, Caesarean section and its indications and risks, and the need for close fetal monitoring are essential before the woman makes an informed choice.

2.16 Management of labour

1 G

Intermittent auscultation is adequate for fetal monitoring.

2 B

LSCS as labour obstruction is imminent. Malpositions are common in parous women. Care should be taken before augmenting labour.

3 C

Expectant management is the choice as there is no fetal compromise.

4 K

Delivery of the second twin in case of descent of the head into the pelvis includes oxytocin and artificial rupture of membranes with continuous fetal heart monitoring.

2.17 Multiple pregnancy

1   O

Two to three weekly routine fetal ultrasound assessments are recommended for monochorionic twin gestation.

2   C

Increased risk of preterm labour indicates steroid administration.

3   O

Small for dates is more common in twin gestation. Reassurance and 2–3 weekly growth scans are recommended once IUGR is noted.

4   D

Triplet pregnancy may include a monochorionic pair and increased vigilance is required.
(See further: *Management of Monochorionic Twin Pregnancy. Green-top Guideline No. 51.* December 2008)

2.18 Assisted vaginal delivery

1   G

Duration of second stage may be longer than 2 hours if other maternal and fetal parameters are normal and delivery is imminent.

2   L

Vacuum delivery is contraindicated in preterm labour.

3   B

Two unsuccessful attempts warrant immediate delivery with a Caesarean section.

4   L

Outlet forceps is the choice of instrument because of thrombocytopenia, when an imminent second-stage delivery needs to be expedited.
(See further: *SOGC Clinical Practice. Guideline No. 148*. August 2004)

2.19 Intrauterine fetal demise

1   **E**

Expectant management: risk to the surviving twin of death or neurological abnormality is in the order of 12% and 18%, respectively.
(See further: *Management of Monochorionic Twin Pregnancy. Green-top Guideline No. 51.* December 2008)

2   **D**

Immediate offer to call her partner, relatives or friends is made. Counselling the patient and other family members is the first step in management. While safety must be assured, medical management should not be rushed.

3   **J**

A combination of mifepristone and a prostaglandin preparation should usually be recommended as the first-line intervention for induction of labour.
(See further: *Green-top Guideline No. 55.* October 2010)

4   **B**

Placental abruption and potential complications like DIC need to be considered.

5   **G**

Initial correction of metabolic and coagulation status followed by obstetric management.

2.20 Psychiatric disease in pregnancy and puerperium

1   C

Fluoxetine is a selective serotonin reuptake inhibitor (SSRI), which increases serotonin neurotransmission and has the lowest known risk during pregnancy. She is safe to continue this.

2   L

Involvement of a psychiatric team is important before commencing treatment.

3   H

Women who need inpatient care for a mental health problem within 12 months of childbirth should normally be admitted to a special mother and baby unit unless there are specific reasons for not doing so.

4   F

Postnatal blues are extremely common and good counselling is the essential first step in the management.

5   F

Post-traumatic stress disorder needs extensive counselling (high-intensity psychological intervention).
(See further: *Antenatal and Postnatal Mental Health: Clinical Management and Service Guidance. NICE Guidelines* [CG192]. Published: December 2014; updated: June 2015)

2.21 Surgical problems/abdominal pain in pregnancy

1   **D**

Severe gastritis is the most likely diagnosis.

2   **G**

Uterine incarceration is a rare complication with a retroverted uterus. The incidence is about 1/3000 pregnancies. It happens usually between 12 and 14 weeks gestation.

3   **A**

Acute appendicitis.

4   **O**

Acute pyelonephritis is characterised by the presence of fever, flank pain and tenderness.

5   **K**

Red degeneration of fibroid is managed conservatively with hydration and good analgesia.

2.22 Impaired glucose metabolism in pregnancy

1   **D**

Folic acid supplementation along with diet and exercise advice.

2   **H**

Immediate treatment with insulin with or without metformin as well as diet advice is considered for fasting plasma glucose level between 6.0 and 6.9 mmol/L if there are additional complications such as macrosomia or hydramnios.

3   **K**

Induction of labour. Induction or Caesarean section (if indicated) should be offered to women with type 1 or type 2 diabetes at 37–38 weeks gestation.

4   **L**

OGTT test with 75 g glucose and 2 hours sugar test is offered as early screening. (See further: *Diabetes in Pregnancy: Management from Preconception to the Postnatal Period. NICE Guidelines [NG3].* Published: February 2015; updated: August 2015)

2.23 Antepartum haemorrhage

1   **F**

Excessive show/vaginal bleeding is an indication for continuous fetal heart monitoring.

2   **I**

Abruption is the most likely diagnosis and immediate resuscitative efforts are required.

3   **A**

Amniotomy rules out abruption and helps in augmenting labour.

4   **B**

Steroids for fetal lung maturity and observation is required.

2.24 Respiratory diseases in pregnancy

1   G

Acute severe asthma is an emergency and should be treated vigorously in the hospital. Immediate nebulisation with oxygen and beta agonists followed by prevention of further episodes need to be considered.

2   E

CT pulmonary angiogram is the gold standard for diagnosing pulmonary embolism.

3   K

Nutritional (iron deficiency) anaemia is the most common pathology.

4   F

Pneumonia has serious implications and immediate hospitalisation and supportive care is required.

2.25 Risk management in obstetrics

1   H

Incident reporting is part of clinical governance. Further obstetric management should be initiated after good counselling. Unexplained IUD is a trigger for incident reporting.

2   G

Initial resuscitation and high dependency care is the first step in management.

3   J

After initial management, root cause analysis with primary physician team, community care team and social services needs to be done. The reason for inadequate interpretation at booking visit and failure to communicate before term need to be explored.

4   C

Good counselling about the entire events and future implications to the patient and family in a sensitive way is the key in managing the patient.

2.26 Intrauterine growth restriction

1   **M**

Reassurance and serial growth scans are recommended.

2   **H**

More than two risk factors such as BMI and age along with a low PAPP-A warrant low-dose aspirin.

3   **A**

Fetal karyotyping to rule out chromosomal defects is recommended.

4   **G**

Immediate delivery LSCS with good neonatal support is indicated.
(See further: *The Investigation and Management of the Small-for-gestational-age Fetus. Green-top Guideline No. 31*, 2nd Edition, February 2013; updated: January 2014)

2.27 Haematological diseases in pregnancy

1   J

Iron deficiency or anaemia due to poor nutrition is the likely possibility.

2   C

Pancytopenia needs immediate evaluation and treatment due to the risks of bleeding and infection.

3   I

Thrombocytopenia most probably idiopathic in origin needs to be considered. However, it is a diagnosis of exclusion.

4   G

HELLP syndrome is the most dreaded situation in severe pre-eclampsia, which might lead to DIC.

Chapter 3: Gynaecology EMQs

3.1 Urogynaecology

Options:

A bladder diary
B blood culture
C post-void residual urine test
D cystoscopy and bladder biopsy
E referral under 2-week rule
F symptom questionnaire
G ultrasound of the renal tract
H urinalysis
I urine culture and sensitivity
J urine cytology
K urine staining and culture for fungus
L urodynamics

For each of the following questions, choose an appropriate investigation option from the list A–L. Each response may be chosen once, more than once or not at all.

Questions:

1   A 30-year-old woman presents to the gynaecology outpatient department (OPD) with a 6-month history of urinary urgency – frequency but no urge incontinence or nocturia. The GP letter states that the urinalysis done last fortnight reported negative.

2   A 72-year-old woman presents to the GP with presence of blood in her urine over the last 2 months. She has no fever or any other systemic symptoms. Routine urinalysis shows blood 3+. She feels quite well and has been brought to the GP reluctantly by her persuasive daughter. The patient apologises for being an encumbrance.

3   A 41-year-old woman presents with a long history of probable recurrent urinary tract infections and has been treated with presumptive antibiotics when she lived abroad. She has severe pain in the bladder area and also urinary urgency but no leaks. She also reports occasional haematuria that resolves spontaneously. Serial urine cultures have always been negative, including for fungus and atypical bacteria.

4   A 38-year-old woman presents with urinary leakage on coughing and sneezing. She has completed her family. She has had two normal deliveries. She also admits that she has difficulty holding on due to urinary urgency and frequents the toilet at least seven times a day but not at night. Anticholinergics have not been helpful so far.

For answers, see 4.1.

3.2 Adolescent gynaecology

Options:

A haematocolpos
B hypothalamic pituitary ovarian axis immaturity
C lower genital tract agenesis
D Mccune–Albright's syndrome
E MRKH (Mayer–Rokitansky–Küster–Hauser) syndrome
F ovarian agenesis
G pelvic actinomycosis
H Sheehan's syndrome
I testicular feminisation syndrome
J Turner's syndrome
K uterus didelphys, dicolpos

For each of the following questions, choose an appropriate diagnosis option from the list A–K. Each response may be chosen once, more than once or not at all.

Questions:

1 A 17-year-old girl is brought to the gynaecology outpatient department with a history of primary amenorrhoea. On questioning, she admits to having cyclical abdominal pain and increasing difficulty with, not in voiding urine and defecation.

2 A 21-year-old patient presents to the gynaecology OPD with complaints of not having periods after her premature delivery of twins 15 months ago. She did not have lactation at all, and the baby has been fed with formula milk throughout. Her GP has recently recommended a thyroxine supplementation due to her weight gain and abnormal thyroid results. She mentions that she does not like coffee anymore as she cannot perceive, not bear its aroma.

3 A 19-year-old girl presents to the GP with intermittent lower abdominal pain and persistent vaginal discharge with no itching or foul smell. She mentions that she is nulliparous and uses an IUD for contraception. It was inserted a year ago.

4 An 18-year-old girl presents to the OPD with cessation of her period that commenced at 15 years of age. It has been increasingly infrequent over the last 2 years and she has not had a period for more than a year now. On examination, it was found that she has a wide carrying angle.

For answers, see 4.2.

3.3 Disorders of menstrual bleeding

Options:

A   cervical punch biopsy
B   chlamydia screening
C   colposcopy-guided biopsy
D   complete blood count
E   dilatation and curettage
F   endocervical curettage
G   endometrial biopsy – Pipelle
H   hysteroscopy and biopsy
I   pap smear
J   reassurance
K   transvaginal ultrasound of the pelvis
L   ultrasound of the abdomen

For each of the following questions, choose an appropriate management option from the list A–L. Each response may be chosen once, more than once or not at all.

Questions:

1   A 13-year-old girl is brought to the gynaecology OPD by her mother. Her mother is concerned that she has not had her periods regularly. She attained menarche at 12 years and had been having periods once in 2 months or sometimes 3 months. She has a normal BMI and plays sport regularly.

2   A 23-year-old university student presents to the gynaecology OPD with prolonged bleeding lasting for 8 days during her period, although not particularly heavy. On questioning, she admits to having intermenstrual and post-coital bleeding intermittently. She uses the combined oral contraceptive pill for contraception.

3   A 40-year-old woman who has recently come from Turkey presents with intermenstrual bleeding. She has not had any investigations so far.

4   A 54-year-old woman presents with spotting of blood vaginally on wiping over the last few weeks on and off. She went through the menopause 3 years ago and is otherwise well. She is more active since her recent knee replacement surgery. Her Pap smear 2 years ago was normal as were her other smears.

For answers, see 4.3.

3.4 Premenstrual syndrome

Options:

A   analgesia
B   CBT
C   Cerazette
D   COC pill with cyproterone
E   COC pill with drospirenone
F   danazol
G   GnRH analogue
H   minipill
I   pyridoxine
J   spironolactone
K   selective serotonin reuptake inhibitor
L   thiamine
M   total abdominal hysterectomy with bilateral salpingo-oophorectomy

For each of the following questions, choose an appropriate treatment option from the list A–M. Each response may be chosen once, more than once or not at all.

Questions:

1   An 18-year-old girl presents to the gynaecology clinic with severe mood swings and delay for a week before the onset of her period. She also feels drained due to heavy bleeding during her periods. This affects her relationship with her boyfriend with whom she is in a stable cohabiting relationship. It also affects her University performance as a new student.

2   A 24-year-old woman presents to the gynaecology clinic with painful periods. She takes a fibre supplement for managing constipation. She also mentions that her GP specifically asked her to discuss her repeated need to see the GP about low mood lasting a week or fortnight that gets better after she has the period pain. The GP had advised her to see a counsellor, but she is not keen to discuss this with anyone else.

3   A 39-year-old woman presents with severe puffiness of the feet and bloating 10 days before her period every month. Her weight increases marginally and she struggles to fit into her well-fitted clothes periodically. She works as a stewardess and finds it distressing. She has no mood changes to report.

4   A 43-year-old woman presents to the gynaecology OPD with complaints of severe mood swings prior to her 24-day cycle lasting more than a week. This is very recent, and she admits to worsening of mood cyclically, but work has also been stressful of late. She explains that she feels a total lack of control and is prone to episodes of feeling tearful. She wants to know if this is due to her hormonal cyclical changes or work stress alone.

For answers, see 4.4.

3.5 Subfertility

Options:

A antral follicle count on transvaginal ultrasound
B hysterosalpingogram
C hysteroscopy
D laparoscopic assessment
E luteal phase progesterone
F semenalysis
G serum antisperm antibodies
H serum estradiol
I serum FSH
J serum LH
K serum prolactin
L serum thyroid-stimulating hormone

For each of the following questions, choose an appropriate management option from the list A–L. Each response may be chosen once, more than once or not at all.

Questions:

1   A 30-year-old woman and her partner present to the subfertility clinic anxious to conceive. They have been trying for a pregnancy for 2 years now. The woman has regular cycles with normal BMI and no prior medical illness. Semenalysis shows a volume of 2 mL with a count of 4 million/mL and 5% normal forms; 35% have progressive motility.

2   A 27-year-old woman presents to the fertility clinic with secondary subfertility. She has a 7-year-old child born of normal conception and had a normal delivery. She has ever used only male condom for contraception. Her cycles have been regular until a year ago. She gets very slight bleeding and has not had a period for 3 months. She complains of vague headache and difficulty in looking out of the corner of both her eyes. Urine pregnancy test is negative in the clinic today.

3   A 32-year-old woman presents to the fertility clinic with primary subfertility. Her periods are regular and her husband's semenalysis is reported to be normal. She undergoes a hysterosalpingogram, which shows filling of the uterine cavity but no further progression of the dye beyond both cornua.

4   A 30-year-old man presents to the fertility clinic with his partner to discuss about starting a family. He admits to being HIV positive and is very compliant with his medications and is under follow-up with the local sexual health service team. His viral load is found to be 30 copies per mL recently. The woman is 26 years old and has regular cycles and has had a child in her previous relationship.

For answers, see 4.5.

3.6 Ectopic pregnancy

Options:

A airway, breathing and circulation assessment
B expectant management
C intramuscular methotrexate
D intratubal methotrexate
E laparoscopic salpingectomy
F laparoscopic salpingotomy
G laparoscopic salpingostomy
H open salpingectomy
I open salpingotomy
J serum progesterone
K ultrasound guided methotrexate into the sac

For each of the following questions, choose an appropriate management option from the list A–K. Each response may be chosen once, more than once or not at all.

Questions:

1 A 25-year-old woman presents with 6-week amenorrhoea and severe lower abdominal pain and tenesmus. Urine pregnancy test is positive in A and E and an ultrasound shows the presence of a sac in the left adnexa and free fluid in the pelvis and an empty uterine cavity. She tolerates the scan poorly due to tenderness. The beta-hCG is reported to be 5400 IU. She is hemodynamically stable.

2 A 30-year-old woman presents to the early pregnancy unit with mild spotting PV and abdominal pain at 8-week gestation. The pregnancy test is positive. The ultrasound reveals an adnexal mass of 8 mm by 4 mm alongside the right ovary. There is no free fluid. The beta-hCG is 150 IU.

3 A 26-year-old presents in her first pregnancy at 7-week gestation with lower abdominal pain and spotting. She has had a beta-hCG 2 days ago that was 900 IU. Her transvaginal scan today shows a very low gestational sac with good Doppler flow beyond the internal os with no sliding sign. A repeat beta-hCG today is 1118 IU.

For answers, see 4.6.

3.7 Management of miscarriage

Options:

A expectant management
B intravaginal misoprostol 200 mg
C intravaginal misoprostol 600 mg
D intravaginal misoprostol 800 mg
E local potassium chloride
F methotrexate
G mifepristone
H oral misoprostol 600 mg
I repeat transvaginal ultrasound
J serum beta-hCG
K urine beta-hCG after 3 weeks

For each of the following questions, choose the most appropriate management option from the list A–K. Each response may be chosen once, more than once or not at all.

Questions:

1 A 24-year-old woman presents with moderate vaginal bleeding with crampy abdominal pain at 6-week gestation. Her urine pregnancy test was positive 10 days ago. Speculum examination shows a partially open cervix. A transvaginal ultrasound shows an open internal os with mixed echoes within the cervical canal. There is a small gestational sac with yolk sac and sliding sign is positive.

2 A 37-year-old woman returns for her review to the early pregnancy unit. She was noted to have an incomplete miscarriage a week ago. Her bleeding has gradually tailed off over the week. On examination, it was found that the os is closed and there is no vaginal bleeding.

3 A 34-year-old woman presents to the GP with spotting at 9-week gestation. She is referred to the early pregnancy unit where she is found to have a missed miscarriage.

4 You are reviewing the histology results for your consultant. Mrs. X, 32-year-old with a missed miscarriage and empty gestation sac, opted to have a suction evacuation. Histology of the products of conception shows a decidual reaction with absence of chorionic villi.

For answers, see 4.7.

3.8 Management of ovarian cysts

Options:

A   AFP, LDH and hCG
B   Ca 125
C   combined oral contraceptive pill
D   expectant management
E   further imaging with MRI
F   IOTA scoring
G   laparoscopic removal of cyst
H   laparoscopic removal of ovary
I   laparotomy
J   laparotomy and ovarian cystectomy
K   progesterone only pill
L   repeat ultrasound
M   RMI
N   TAH and BSO
O   ultrasound-guided aspiration

For each of the following questions, choose the most appropriate management option from the list A–O. Each response may be chosen once, more than once or not at all.

Questions:

1   A 26-year-old woman presents to the gynaecology OPD with an ultrasound scan of her pelvis for menorrhagia. It reports an anechoic ovarian cyst of 28 mm × 37 mm on the right side. No other abnormal findings are reported.

2   A 54-year-old woman presents with abdominal pain and has had an ultrasound scan done. It showed an ovarian cyst which triggered a transvaginal scan. Pain has resolved now. A 46-mm cyst with a thin wall within with normal CA 125 is noted. She has a repeat scan after 2 months that shows a 58 mm cyst with similar features and normal tumour markers. No new symptoms are noted.

3   A 60-year-old woman has an ultrasound scan done for non-specific abdominal pain and is found to have an ovarian cyst of 28 mm which is fluid filled. The Ca 125 is normal and the RMI is 100. She is advised a further scan after 4 months. The cyst has not changed in nature and the size is 22 mm.

For answers, see 4.8.

3.9 Abdominal pain

Options:

A   acute appendicitis
B   ectopic pregnancy
C   endometriosis
D   functional pain
E   haemorrhage into ovarian cyst
F   Meckel's diverticulitis
G   mid-cyclical pain
H   Mittelschmerz
I   ovarian cyst rupture
J   ovarian torsion
K   pelvic inflammatory disease
L   urinary tract infection

For each of the following questions, choose the most appropriate diagnosis from the list A–L. Each response may be chosen once, more than once or not at all.

Questions:

1   A 23-year-old woman presents with lower abdominal pain which is bilateral. She has diffuse tenderness on examination, is febrile and her period was 3 weeks ago. A urine pregnancy test is negative. Speculum examination reveals a congested cervix and cervical excitation.

2   A 22-year-old woman is brought to the Accident and Emergency department with complaints of diarrhoea with sudden onset of abdominal pain and fainting spell. She uses the minipill but is noncompliant. She has irregular periods.

3   A 24-year-old woman is brought to the hospital with complaints of abdominal pain and spotting. Her period was 2 weeks ago, and the pregnancy test is negative. She is afebrile, has no gastrointestinal symptoms, examination is normal and recovers with simple analgesia.

4   A 25-year-old woman presents to the hospital with abdominal pain and vomiting. She had nausea for more than 24 hours. She is pyrexial and has tenderness with cervical movement. Urine pregnancy test is negative.

For answers, see 4.9.

3.10 Menopausal symptoms

Options:

A   alendronate
B   black cohosh
C   clonidine
D   cognitive behavioural therapy
E   estrogen and progesterone continuous combined hormone replacement therapy (HRT)
F   estrogen and progesterone cyclical oral hormone replacement
G   estrogen only oral hormone replacement
H   ginseng
I   isoflavone
J   progesterone only hormone therapy
K   SNRI
L   SSRI
M   testosterone hormone therapy
N   tibolone
O   vaginal estrogen gel
P   vaginal estrogen tablet

For each of the following questions, choose the most appropriate management option from the list A–P. Each response may be chosen once, more than once or not at all.

Questions:

1   A 52-year-old woman presents with complaints of low libido. She attained menopause 5 years ago and is taking estrogen and progesterone HRT.

2   A 56-year-old woman presents to the urogynaecology clinic with dysuria and vaginal irritation. This has been a problem for many months. Urine routine and culture are negative for bacterial presence. Local examination shows a urethral caruncle.

3   A 52-year-old woman presents with severe hot flushes. She takes tablets for hypertension that has been well managed for the past 6 years. She had a hysterectomy when she was 49.

4   A 48-year-old woman presents with amenorrhoea for 10 months. She is concerned about her family history of osteoporosis and a recent DEXA scan showed a low T score with osteopenia globally. Her mum and aunt have been operated for breast cancer.

For answers, see 4.10.

3.11 Polycystic ovarian syndrome

Options:

A   Cerazette
B   combined oral contraceptive pill with cyproterone
C   combined oral contraceptive pill with drospirenone
D   metformin
E   orlistat
F   ovarian drilling
G   progesterone only pill
H   reassurance
I   regular gestogen withdrawal bleeding
J   weight loss

For each of the following questions, choose the most appropriate management option from the list A–J. Each response may be chosen once, more than once or not at all.

Questions:

1   A 13-year-old girl is brought to the gynaecology OPD by her mother. She attained menarche a year ago but has had only two cycles in the year. She weighs 48 kg. Her BMI is normal. The mother is concerned as she has polycystic ovary syndrome (PCOS).

2   A 24-year-old woman presents to the gynaecology OPD with irregular periods. She has a 6-month history of amenorrhoea. Her periods have been irregular for the last 2 years. She is not in a relationship currently. She has been advised weight loss by the GP and is trying to maintain a healthy diet and active lifestyle.

3   A 35-year-old woman with a BMI of 22 presents to the fertility clinic. She has irregular cycles once in 2–3 months and is anxious to conceive. Her ultrasound reveals polycystic ovaries.

4   A 32-year-old parous woman presents to the gynaecology clinic as she is unable to lose weight. She was diagnosed with PCOS but has never had any menstrual irregularity.

For answers, see 4.11.

3.12 Female genital mutilation

Options:

A   assess in labour
B   counsel about illegal nature of act
C   deinfibulation
D   elective anterior episiotomy in labour
E   elective division of scar tissue before onset of labour
F   inform police
G   inform specialist midwife
H   local examination for assessment
I   reassurance
J   refer to plastic surgery
K   refer to social services
L   reinfibulation

For each of the following questions, choose the most appropriate management option from the list A–L. Each response may be chosen once, more than once or not at all.

Questions:

1   A 17-year-old woman presents to the gynaecology OPD with abdominal pain. She has recently relocated to England and has a 6-month-old child delivered by Caesarean section. Examination reveals a type 3 female genital mutilation (FGM).

2   A 28-year-old woman presents to the gynaecology OPD with painful periods. She is accompanied by her 12-year-old daughter. The mother informs that they are about to travel to their home country for traditional 'private surgery' of the 12-year-old girl as it is illegal in the United Kingdom to do so.

3   A 32-year-old woman visits the gynaecology clinic after her first childbirth. She was noted to have type 1 FGM in labour and needed division of the scar in labour prior to childbirth. She requests a reinfibulation.

4   An antenatal woman books late in pregnancy at 25 weeks gestation as she moved into the country only 2 months ago. During the booking visit, she mentions that she has had FGM as a child. Examination in antenatal clinic reveals a type 2 infibulation. The urethra is visible and she has had a Pap smear 2 years ago when she was a student in the United Kingdom.

For answers, see 4.12.

3.13 Cervical screening I

Options:

A   endometrial sampling
B   local antibacterial wash
C   reassurance
D   remove IUCD if asymptomatic
E   sitz bath
F   treat with clindamycin
G   treat with clotrimazole ointment
H   treat with clotrimazole pessary
I   treat with erythromycin
J   treat with metronidazole orally
K   treat with oral fluconazole
L   vaginal douching

For each of the following questions, choose the most appropriate management option from the list A–L. Each response may be chosen once, more than once or not at all.

Questions:

1   A 36-year-old woman undergoes routine cervical screening. She has no gynaecological problems. An IUCD is seen. The report is negative for cervical intraepithelial neoplasia and actinomyces-like organisms (ALOs) are seen.

2   A 29-year-old woman has a routine smear with the GP. She has no gynaecological symptoms. The report is negative for cervical intraepithelial neoplasia, but *Candida* spores are noted during microscopy.

3   A 46-year-old woman presents to her GP surgery for a routine cervical smear with the nurse. Her smear is reported negative for cervical intraepithelial neoplasia and some clue cells have been reported on microscopy.

4   A 33-year-old woman presents to a community clinic for cervical screening. Her last menstrual period was 8 days ago. Her report is negative for cervical intraepithelial neoplasia with the presence of endometrial cells.

5   A 45-year-old woman presents to a community clinic for cervical screening. Her last menstrual period was 12 days ago. Her report is negative for cervical intraepithelial neoplasia with clusters of endometrial cells.

For answers, see 4.13.

3.14 Cervical screening II

Options:

A   two-week referral to colposcopy
B   two-week referral to gynaecology clinic
C   LLETZ under general anaesthesia
D   LLETZ under local anaesthetic block
E   routine recall
F   no further Pap smears
G   repeat smear with GP after 6 months
H   routine referral to colposcopy in 6 weeks
I   see and treat colposcopy in 2 weeks
J   test of cure – High-risk HPV DNA
K   test of triage – High-risk HPV DNA test

For each of the following questions, choose the most appropriate management option from the list A–K. Each response may be chosen once, more than once or not at all.

Questions:

1   A 26-year-old woman undergoes her first cervical routine screening test. Her smear is reported as borderline squamous cell changes.

2   A 26-year-old patient has had a routine smear which revealed borderline squamous cell changes on cytology. She has had a high-risk HPV DNA test that has been reported to be positive.

3   A 34-year-old woman has a routine smear test that has revealed a low-grade dyskaryosis. She has a test of triage which has been reported to be negative.

4   A 50-year-old woman undergoes her routine cervical screening. The results are reported as high-grade moderate dyskaryosis.

For answers, see 4.14.

3.15 Cervical screening III

Options:

A two-week referral to colposcopy
B two-week referral to gynaecology clinic
C LLETZ under general anaesthesia
D LLETZ under local anaesthetic block
E no further Pap smears
F repeat smear with GP after 6 months
G routine recall
H routine referral to colposcopy in 6 weeks
I see and treat colposcopy in 2 weeks
J test of cure – High-risk HPV DNA
K test of triage – High-risk HPV DNA test

For each of the following questions, choose the most appropriate management option from the list A–K. Each response may be chosen once, more than once or not at all.

Questions:

1 A 52-year-old woman presents to her GP surgery for a repeat smear as her previous routine smear 6 months ago was inadequate. The second sample now has been reported as inadequate too.

2 A 37-year-old woman presents to the clinic for her routine smear. The report reads as follows: CGIN, endocervical cells with changes of CGIN seen.

3 A 40-year-old woman has her routine smear at the Community Gynaecology clinic. The smear is reported as borderline dyskaryosis.

4 A 43-year-old woman has a routine Pap smear. It is reported negative for cervical cell dyskaryosis. However, endometrial clusters of cells are noted. Her last menstrual period was 10 days ago, and she has regular periods.

For answers, see 4.15.

3.16 Risk of complications in abdominal hysterectomy for benign reasons

Options:

A 1 in 100
B 2 in 100
C 4 in 100
D 7 in 100
E 15 in 100
F 23 in 100
G 1 in 1000
H 2 in 1000
I 4 in 1000
J 7 in 1000
K 15 in 1000
L 23 in 1000

For each of the following questions, choose the most appropriate counselling risk to be mentioned for a benign abdominal hysterectomy from the list A–L. Each response may be chosen once, more than once or not at all.

Questions:

1 The overall risk of the patient having any complication after such surgery.

2 The risk of damage to the urinary system, including the ureter and the bladder, and the long-term urinary dysfunction.

3 Loss of blood requiring a blood transfusion.

4 Return to theatre due to bleeding, wound dehiscence or such complications.

5 Thromboembolic event comprising deep vein thrombosis and pulmonary thromboembolism.

For answers, see 4.16.

3.17 Risks following repair of obstetric anal sphincter injury

Options:

A   1 in 100
B   6 in 100
C   8 in 100
D   9 in 100
E   16 in 100
F   18 in 100
G   26 in 100
H   28 in 100
I   36 in 100
J   38 in 100

For each of the following questions, choose the most appropriate counselling risk to be mentioned after a repair of obstetric anal sphincter injury from the list A–J. Each response may be chosen once, more than once or not at all.

Questions:

1   An overwhelming desire to pass stools.

2   Pain in the perineum or during intercourse.

3   Sepsis at the site of the sphincter repair.

For answers, see 4.17.

3.18 Long-acting reversible contraception failure

Options:

A   1 per 1000
B   4 per 1000
C   8 per 1000
D   10 per 1000
E   14 per 1000
F   18 per 1000
G   20 per 1000
H   24 per 1000
I   28 per 1000
J   30 per 1000

For each of the following questions, choose the most appropriate management option from the list A–J. Each response may be chosen once, more than once or not at all.

Questions:

1   A 30-year-old woman has had two normal deliveries. Her last childbirth was 6 months ago. Her period is regular and is requesting a non-hormonal intrauterine contraceptive device. She wishes to know the failure of the copper IUCD.

2   A 40-year-old woman has an 8-year-old girl and wishes to have an efficient contraceptive method. She has heavy periods and is counselled for a progesterone IUS. She requests to know the failure of the progesterone IUS.

3   A 26-year-old nulliparous woman is in a stable relationship. She has been taking the minipill due to her migraines and wishes to have an injectable progesterone as she sometimes forgets to take the pill. She requests information about the reliability of the method as a contraceptive.

4   A 30-year-old nulliparous woman presents to the family planning services to seek some information about contraception choices. She wishes to know about a long-acting contraceptive with the lowest risk of failure and is reversible.

For answers, see 4.18.

Chapter 4: Gynaecology Answers

4.1 Urogynaecology

1   **A**

A bladder diary helps to ascertain the type and quantity of the ingested fluids and the association with urinary symptoms. As she does not have urinary leakage, dry overactive bladder may be managed with a symptom diary for confirmation of diagnosis and patient feedback with lifestyle recommendations before commencing medications.

2   **E**

Presence of blood in the urine with no suggestion of urinary infection is a worrying symptom that needs an immediate referral to the secondary care. Some units have a dedicated haematuria clinic for this purpose.

3   **D**

The symptoms are suggestive of interstitial cystitis. Cystoscopy and a probable biopsy will help in the diagnosis. These patients are often mistaken for overactive bladder or recurrent UTI.

4   **L**

Urodynamics helps to ascertain treatment plan if conservative measures have not been helpful.

4.2 Adolescent gynaecology

1   A

Non-canalisation of the lowermost end of the urogenital tract in women may lead to haematocolpos. Improper ectodermal development or derangement in canalisation may lead to this condition. Examination reveals a bulge due to accumulated menstrual blood.

2   H

Sheehan's post-partum pituitary necrosis happens due to diminished blood supply to the thalamus after a post-partum haemorrhage if adequate fluid replacement is delayed. It manifests as pituitary dysfunction with multiple endocrine problems, including anosmia and thyroid dysfunction.

3   G

Pelvic actinomycosis is associated with symptoms of irregular bleeding discharge, abdominal pain and sometimes a pelvic mass. This can be treated with specific antibiotics usually. Persistent symptomatic infection may need removal of the IUCD.

4   J

Turner's syndrome can lead to early ovarian failure. Premature destruction of oocytes occurs due to the presence of the 45×0 chromosome type.

4.3 Disorders of menstrual bleeding

1   J

Reassurance as irregular cycles are common in the initial few months or years after menarche. There is no need for intervention unless the cycles are excessively heavy or painful.

2   B

Screening for chlamydia is helpful. Irregular bleeding pattern in young women who are sexually active is often due to chlamydia infection.

3   I

Pap smear and cervical inspection is the first stage in the investigation of abnormal bleeding. Many countries outside the United Kingdom do not have a routine cervical screening programme.

4   K

Transvaginal ultrasound helps to exclude endometrial pathology. Obesity and association with immobility are not uncommon.

4.4 Premenstrual syndrome

1   E

Premenstrual syndrome in adolescence with a need for contraception and treatment of menorrhagia may benefit from a combined oral contraceptive pill containing drospirenone.

2   K

Severe mood swings may be managed using an SSRI such as citalopram.

3   J

Spironolactone is an effective measure. It is a potassium-sparing diuretic that may be helpful particularly with water retention prior to periods.

4   G

Gonadotropin-releasing hormone analogues help to a certain extent by blocking the gonadotropin hormones. Any cyclical changes alone will improve with this intervention.

(See further: *GTG on premenstrual syndrome*)

4.5 Subfertility

1   F

Repeat semenalysis is advised with a single abnormal test preferably after 3 months. World Health Organization reference values:

- Semen volume: 1.5 mL or more
- pH: 7.2 or more
- Sperm concentration: 15 million spermatozoa per mL or more
- Total sperm number: 39 million spermatozoa per ejaculate or more
- Total motility (percentage of progressive motility and non-progressive motility): 40% or more motile or 32% or more with progressive motility
- Vitality: 58% or more live spermatozoa
- Sperm morphology (percentage of normal forms): 4% or more

2   K

Serum prolactin is likely to be elevated with anovulation and possible bitemporal hemianopia. Galactorrhoea may be associated.

3   D

Laparoscopic assessment of the tubes is required to ascertain the findings and the level of damage along with a complete pelvic assessment.

4   F

Semenalysis to find if the parameters are normal. Unprotected intercourse for conception around the period of fertility with viral load less than 50 copies/mL is recommended.
(See further: *NICE Guidance CG 156*)

4.6 Ectopic pregnancy

1 **F**

Laparoscopic salpingectomy is advised if an ectopic pregnancy is found on laparoscopy and the patient has acute bleeding loss into the peritoneal cavity. The contralateral tube is checked to ensure that it appears normal during the laparoscopy.

2 **B**

Expectant management with serial beta-hCG and follow-up until complete decline is advised with low levels of beta-hCG.

3 **C**

The clinical history points towards a cervical ectopic pregnancy. Systemic methotrexate is currently found to be more useful (91% of patients). (See further: *GTG- Ectopic Pregnancy Management*)

4.7 Management of miscarriage

1 **A**

Expectant management of the situation is advisable. If the bleeding is not heavy and the clinical findings are suggestive of a miscarriage, conservative management may be followed. The presence of yolk sac confirms the intrauterine gestation, and sliding sign excludes a cervical ectopic pregnancy.

2 **K**

In the absence of bleeding or signs of infection, a repeat ultrasound is not necessary in a spontaneous miscarriage. However, a 3-week urine pregnancy test will complete the follow-up.

3 **C**

Intravaginal misoprostol 800 mg is advised after a missed miscarriage to expedite expulsion of products of conception.

4 **J**

Serum beta-hCG will ensure that this is not an ectopic pregnancy or pregnancy of unknown location with a pseudo-gestational sac.
(See further: *NICE Guidance on Early Pregnancy CG 154*)

4.8 Management of ovarian cysts

1 D

Asymptomatic, incidental, fluid-filled ovarian cysts less than 50 mm do not warrant further imaging or intervention.

2 G

While it is safe to manage an ovarian cyst conservatively when fluid-filled, the increasing size of the cyst needs to be given due concern. It is unlikely to be functional and a laparoscopic cystectomy should be considered.

3 D

Asymptomatic ovarian cysts that do not increase in size with a normal Ca 125 may be managed conservatively.
(See further: *GTG 34 Management of Post-menopausal Ovarian Cysts*)

4.9 Abdominal pain

1   K

Pelvic inflammatory disease should be thought of in the absence of a positive pregnancy test with these symptoms. Culture for gonorrhoea and chlamydia will clinch the diagnosis.

2   B

Ectopic pregnancy must be excluded primarily in any woman with abdominal symptoms in the reproductive age group.

3   H

Mittelschmerz or mid-cyclical pain can be severe and can be disabling in some people.

4   A

Nausea and vomiting occur in most patients with appendicitis, but only 50% of those with PID. Cervical movement pain will occur in about 25% of women with appendicitis. Further blood tests and imaging with ultrasound are helpful in making the diagnosis.
(See further: *BASHH PID Guideline*)

4.10 Menopausal symptoms

1   **M**

Testosterone therapy helps in the alleviation of low libido.

2   **P**

Urogenital symptoms may be severe in some patients after menopause. Local estrogen helps. Vaginal estrogen pessaries are helpful in the alleviation of symptoms.

3   **G**

Estrogen only HRT does not increase additional cardiovascular risk if medical conditions such as hypertension are well managed.

4   **A**

Alendronate is useful in the prevention of osteoporosis with strong family history. A strong family history of breast cancer makes estrogen hormone replacement potentially risky.
(See further: *NICE Guideline 23 – Management of Menopause*)

4.11 Polycystic ovarian syndrome

1   H

Reassure the mother that cycle irregularities are very common after menarche in the first 2 years. However, maintaining a healthy lifestyle is advised. No further investigations need to be undertaken in a young girl of 13 years.

2   I

Regular withdrawal bleeding after 3 months helps to prevent unchecked endometrial growth due to estrogen influence alone. Long-term risk of endometrial hyperplasia is also prevented using progesterone-induced bleeding.

3   F

Laparoscopic ovarian drilling helps to restore ovulation for purposes of conception while checking the tubes and excluding other pelvic pathology.

4   E

Weight loss medications such as orlistat may be helpful in people in whom lifestyle measures have not been of help.
(See further: *GTG Long-term Consequences of PCOS*)

4.12 Female genital mutilation

1   F

A woman under 18 years who had undergone infibulation must be under the care of social services and must be informed to the police within a month of the examination.

2   K

It is illegal to perform the procedure or abet the same. The parent should be counselled against the same. It is mandatory to inform the social services.

3   B

There is no clinical indication for reinfibulation, and the patient should be advised against it.

4   I

If the woman has a visible urethra and Pap smear was possible with a speculum examination, deinfibulation is not essential.
(See further: *GTG Female Genital Mutilation*)

4.13 Cervical screening I

1   C

Asymptomatic ALOs in smear need not be treated.

2   C

The presence of *Candida* on microscopy of the vaginal flora is not an indication for treatment. This is part of the normal vaginal flora and need not be treated in the absence of inflammation on examination or clinical symptoms.

3   J

The presence of clue cells is very specific for bacterial vaginosis and treatment with oral metronidazole is suggested.

4   C

Presence of endometrial cells with a recent period less than 10 days ago and age under 40 years discourages any further tests if asymptomatic.

5   A

Age over 40 years and last menstrual period over 10 days ago are factors that lend significance to the finding. Further endometrial assessment with sampling is essential.
(See further: *NHSCCP Professional Guidelines: Colposcopy Referral*)

4.14 Cervical screening II

1   **K**

A high-risk HPV DNA test is recommended to triage a referral to the colposcopy unit. If negative, she is discharged to routine recall; if positive, she is invited to colposcopy.

2   **H**

A diagnostic colposcopy is recommended.

3   **E**

Low-grade dyskaryosis with negative high-risk DNA test results is reassuring and a routine recall system may be followed.

4   **I**

High-grade smears both moderate and severe are referred to colposcopy under the 2-week rule.
(See further: *NHSCCP Professional Guidelines: Colposcopy Referral*)

4.15 Cervical screening III

1   F

Repeat smear no less than 3 months later is recommended. Three inadequate samples will trigger a referral to colposcopy.

2   I

Referral to colposcopy in 2 weeks is essential for suspected cervical glandular intraepithelial neoplasia.

3   K

A borderline smear should be triaged by the presence of high-risk HPV DNA. A positive test should trigger a referral to colposcopy within 6 weeks.

4   B

Endometrial pathology must be excluded. An urgent referral to the gynaecology clinic is recommended.
(See further: https://www.bsccp.org.uk/assets/file/uploads/resources/ NHSCervicalScreeingProgramme.PublicationNumber20-ThirdEdition.pdf)

4.16 Risk of complications in abdominal hysterectomy for benign reasons

1   C

The risk of a patient having any complication after a benign abdominal hysterectomy is 4 in 100 (common).

2   J

The risk of long-term sequelae or urinary tract injury after hysterectomy is 7 in 1000 (uncommon).

3   L

Enough blood loss warranting a replacement due to hemodynamic compromise is 23 in 1000 (common).

4   J

The risk of return to theatre after an abdominal hysterectomy for benign reasons is 7 in 1000 (uncommon).

5   I

Thromboembolic events are common with a risk of 4 in 1000 (common).
(See further: *RCOG Guidelines, Consent – Abdominal Hysterectomy for Benign Reasons*)

4.17 Risks following repair of obstetric anal sphincter injury

1   G

The risk of faecal urgency is very common in the order of 26 in 100.

2   D

The risk of dyspareunia and perineal pain is common. The risk specified is 9 per 100.

3   C

The risk of wound infection after repair of an obstetric anal sphincter injury is 8 in 100. (See further: *Consent – OASIS, RCOG Guidelines*)

4.18 Long-acting reversible contraception failure

1 **G**

The risk of a copper device with 380 mm^2 of copper is 20 per 1000 in 5 years.

2 **D**

The risk of pregnancy with a progesterone IUS is less than 10 per 1000 in 5 years.

3 **B**

The risk of a pregnancy with the use of an injectable progesterone is very low in the order of 4 per 1000 over 2 years use.

4 **A**

The progesterone etonogestrel implant has a failure rate of 1 per 1000 over a 3-year use. (See further: *NICE CG 30 LARC*)

Recommended Reading List

The recommended reading for candidates for the Part 2 MRCOG exam has been prepared by the RCOG's Part 2 MRCOG Sub-committees.

Books

Bonney's Gynaecological Surgery (11th edition, published 2011)
Tito Lopes, Nick Spirtos, Raj Naik, John M. Monaghan (Wiley)

Clinical Gynecologic Oncology (9th edition, published 2017)
Philip J. DiSaia, William T. Creasman, Robert S. Mannel, D. Scott McMeekin, David G. Mutch (Elsevier)

Contraception: Your Questions Answered (7th edition, published 2017)
John Guillebaud, Anne MacGregor (Elsevier)

Cunningham and Gilstrap's Operative Obstetrics (3rd edition, published 2017)
Edward R. Yeomans, Barbara L. Hoffman, Larry C. Gilstrap III, F. Gary Cunningham (McGraw-Hill)

Dewhurst's Textbook of Obstetrics and Gynaecology (9th edition, published 2012)
D. Keith Edmonds, Christopher Lees, Tom Bourne (Wiley)

Drugs During Pregnancy and Lactation: Treatment Options and Risk Assessment (3rd edition, published 2014)
Christof Schaefer, Paul W.J. Peters, and Richard K. Miller (Academic Press)

Fanaroff and Martin's Neonatal-Perinatal Medicine: Diseases of the Fetus and Infant (10th edition, published 2014)
Richard J. Martin, Avroy A. Fanaroff, Michele C. Walsh (Saunders)

Handbook of Obstetric Medicine (5th edition, published 2015)
Catherine Nelson-Piercy (CRC Press)

High Risk Pregnancy: Management Options (4th edition, published 2011)
David K. James, Philip J. Steer, Carl P. Weiner, Bernard Gonik (Cambridge University Press)

Martindale: The Complete Drug Reference (37th edition, published 2011)
Sean C. Sweetman (Royal Pharmaceutical Society)

RECOMMENDED READING LIST

Obstetrics and Gynaecology: An Evidence-Based Text for MRCOG (3rd edition, published 2016)
David M. Luesley, Mark D. Kilby (CRC Press)

Oxford Speciality Training: Training in Obstetrics & Gynaecology
Ippokratis Sarris, Susan Bewley, Sangeeta Agnihotri (Oxford University Press)

Other resources

- *British National Formulary*
- *NICE Guidelines*
- *RCOG Green-top Guidelines*
- *RCOG Scientific Impact Papers*
- *The Obstetrician & Gynaecologist (TOG)*

Index